To Carrie

From

Much love —

2006

The Miami Mediterranean Diet

Lose Weight and Lower Your Risk of Heart Disease

The healthy, practical and sensible approach based on the clinically proven Mediterranean diet & lifestyle

Michael D. Ozner, M.D.

Cambridge House
Publishing

Cambridge House

P u b l i s h i n g

For further information and bulk purchases:
www.cardiacoz.com
305-596-4545

DISCLAIMER

ISBN 0-9765084-0-0

Library of Congress Control Number: 2005902118

CONTENTS

PART ONE
The Miami Mediterranean Diet and Lifestyle

PART TWO
Recipes

To my wife, Christine,
and my children,
Jennifer and Jonathan:
You are my heart
and soul.

ACKNOWLEDGEMENTS

I would like to thank my patients and colleagues who have given me the inspiration and motivation to write "The Miami Mediterranean Diet".

I am especially grateful to the following colleagues who have taken extensive time and effort to review and critique "The Miami Mediterranean Diet": Barry T. Katzen, M.D., a pioneer in Interventional Radiology and Medical Director of the Baptist Cardiac & Vascular Institute at Baptist Hospital of Miami; Randolph P. Martin, M.D., Director of Noninvasive Cardiology at Emory University in Atlanta; Karen Lieberman, Ph.D., R.D., Professor and Chair of the Hospitality College at Johnson & Wales University, Florida Campus.

I would also like to acknowledge Susan D'Agostino, RN and Lois Exelbert, RN, two nurse educators who share my passion for cardiovascular disease prevention, who have helped me organize and promote the Wellness & Prevention program at the Baptist Cardiac & Vascular Institute at Baptist Hospital of Miami. This program provides education and prevention strategies for patients who have heart disease or diabetes and for those with risk factors for cardiovascular disease.

Finally, I would like to thank my wife, Christine L. Ozner, RN, who has a special interest in nutrition and Mediterranean cooking and has contributed immensely to the writing and editing of this book.

CONGRATULATIONS

*B*y reading this book and following the principles of the Miami Mediterranean diet and lifestyle, you are well on your way of taking charge of your own cardiovascular health. This book is intended to provide information on cardiovascular disease prevention. This book however is not intended to replace the doctor – patient relationship which should exist for all men and women. I recommend that you discuss all prevention and treatment options with your personal treating physician. Regular office visits between the patient and his or her doctor to discuss cardiovascular prevention strategies will provide the optimum approach in the ongoing battle against heart disease.

FOREWORD

*W*e are at war in the United States of America. The enemy is quite formidable. It kills more people than all of the wars we have previously fought. Every 30 seconds it claims another victim. We have identified the enemy but we have not defeated it. Its name is cardiovascular disease.

Is there a solution? Can we defeat cardiovascular disease and its manifestations (heart attack, stroke, peripheral vascular disease)? The answer is yes!

First, we must realize that our most effective weapon is prevention, not intervention. Prevention strategies must begin at an early age and continue for life. Proper diet, exercise, smoking cessation, stress management and medical therapy are the weapons we need in our battle against heart disease.

It is my hope that this book will provide you with the information you need to begin an effective prevention strategy. Don't sit back and wait for this silent killer to strike. Take action before you develop symptoms. I hope you will defeat cardiovascular disease and live a long, happy and heart-healthy life.

INTRODUCTION

*I*t was a typical day for Ted. He awoke at 6am and had his usual breakfast of bacon, eggs and fried potatoes. He left in a hurry after an argument with his wife and drove to his office to begin another stressful day as a real estate executive. At a 9:30 a.m. board meeting, he presented a proposal for purchasing a large office complex. During the meeting he had coffee and doughnuts and smoked several cigarettes. It was customary for Ted to argue with his partners and today was no different. After several phone calls, he was off to the airport to catch a noon flight. He had no time to sit down for lunch, so he drove to his favorite fast food drive-through for a burger and fries, which he quickly ate on the way to the airport. After parking his car and walking briskly to the terminal, he developed crushing chest pain and broke into a sweat. He grabbed a roll of Tums from his pocket and chewed several tablets. The pain subsided, however it returned with a vengeance several minutes later. This time the pain was an intense pressure sensation in his chest which radiated to his arms and his jaw. He had a feeling of impending doom. Ted collapsed at the security gate and lost consciousness. He awoke in a nearby emergency room, having been resuscitated by paramedics. It was clear that Ted suffered a massive heart attack and he was lucky to be alive. Following an extensive hospital stay with heart catheterization and coronary bypass surgery, Ted's life would never be the same.

Giovanni awoke the same day in his small Italian village. He had a light breakfast of bread with jam and fruit. He went to his nearby office and had a pleasant morning with his clients in his import/export business. At 1:30 p.m. he returned home where he had an enjoyable lunch with his family and friends. Lunch consisted of a salad with olive oil, whole wheat pasta, whole grain bread with garlic, goat cheese, red wine and fresh fruit. Following lunch, he rested for an hour and then returned to his business.

Was Ted's heart attack preventable? Is Giovanni's good health a matter of luck? The answer seems crystal clear. A healthy diet along with prudent exercise and relaxation will certainly contribute to a long life of good health. This book will outline the type of diet which this author has used in his practice of cardiology to successfully treat his patients who have had heart attacks or have significant risk factors for cardiovascular disease. This diet is not a fad diet nor one which promises quick weight loss or sensational results. Rather, it is a Mediterranean diet which consists of fresh fruits and vegetables, whole grains, nuts, cheese, olive oil and wine consumed in moderation. This diet encourages consumption of fresh non – processed food and discourages intake of refined sugar, saturated animal fat and preservatives including trans-fats. In fact, this diet is as much a lifestyle as a diet, in which food is shared with family and friends, and exercise and relaxation is encouraged. The health benefits of this type of diet has been proven for centuries in Mediterranean countries.

WAKE UP AMERICA! There is no magical quick fix diet for weight loss or long term health. If one is to embark on a healthy diet and lifestyle then why not choose one that has been proven for hundreds of years. This book will provide you with the information and dietary plan you need to get started on a lifelong journey of healthy eating. Hopefully, by following these guidelines, you will live a long, happy and heart – healthy life.

PART ONE

The Miami Mediterranean Diet and Lifestyle

The Optimal Diet For Cardiovascular Health

I have used the principles of the Mediterranean diet to successfully treat patients in my practice of cardiovascular disease prevention for more than 25 years. Why is the Mediterranean diet the optimal diet for good health and long life? The answer lies in the many clinical trials which have concluded that a Mediterranean diet lowers the risk of heart disease and promotes long term health.

There are many theories which have been postulated to explain the beneficial impact of the Mediterranean diet on heart health, as well as cancer risk. One such theory links saturated fat and trans fat with heart disease and cancer. Consumption of saturated fat and trans fat is limited in the Mediterranean diet.

The Mediterranean diet also decreases inflammation. The role of inflammation in the development and progression of heart disease, cancer and diabetes has been reviewed extensively in the literature. Olive oil, fish and red wine, an integral part of the Mediterranean diet, have been shown to be anti-inflammatory (decreases inflammation). In contrast, the typical American (Western) diet, with a high consumption of saturated fat, trans fat and omega-6 fatty acids, is pro-inflammatory (promotes inflammation).

Below is a summary of the clinical trials that have demonstrated the beneficial impact of Mediterranean diets on our health:

The Seven Countries Study: A landmark 20 year study by Dr. Ancel Keys beginning in the late 1950's demonstrating that a diet low in saturated animal fat and processed food was associated with a low incidence of mortality from coronary heart disease. This study followed almost 13,000 men from seven different countries (Italy, Greece, Yugoslavia, Netherlands, Finland, United States and Japan). The value of eating a Mediterranean diet became clear, as men living in the Mediterranean region had the lowest incidence of heart disease and longest life expectancy in the world. Greek men had a 90% lower likelihood of premature death from heart attack compared to American men!

The Lyon Diet Heart Study: Heart attack survivors placed on a Mediterranean diet was compared to a control diet resembling the American Heart Association Step 1 diet. The Mediterranean diet was associated with a 70% decreased risk of death and a 73% decreased risk of recurrent cardiac events including heart attack and sudden cardiac death. Compared to the American Heart Association Step 1 diet, the Mediterranean diet afforded significantly better protection against recurrent heart attacks and death.

The Singh Study: An Indo-Mediterranean diet rich in fruits, vegetables, whole grains, walnuts & almonds resulted in a significant reduction in serum cholesterol and was associated with a significant reduction in heart attack and sudden cardiac death.

The GISSI - Prevenzion Study: Beginning a Mediterranean diet following a heart attack reduced death rate by 40% over six years. Fish, fruit, vegetables and olive oil all conferred benefit. In addition, taking a fish oil capsule daily decreased the risk of sudden cardiac death by 45%.

The Attica Study: Adherence to the traditional Mediterranean diet was associated with a reduction in the blood markers of inflammation and clotting.

Mediterranean Diet Study: Greater adherence to the traditional Mediterranean diet in more than 22,000 adults in Greece over a period of 44 months was associated with a significant reduction in death due to heart disease and cancer.

The Dart Trial: 32% reduction in coronary heart disease death and a 29% reduction in overall death by consuming oily fish (such as salmon, tuna and sardines) at least twice a week.

Why has the Mediterranean diet lowered the risk of death from heart disease and cancer compared to an American or Western diet? The answer is due to a number of beneficial aspects of this type of diet and lifestyle:

Olive oil

Olive oil is the "soul" of the Mediterranean diet and provides the taste and flavor of Mediterranean dishes. It is made by crushing and then pressing olives. Olive oil is a rich source of monounsaturated fat – the type of fat which is beneficial for heart health. The regular use of olive oil instead of other fats is associated with a reduced risk of heart disease, cancer, diabetes and inflammatory disorders like asthma and arthritis.

Olive oil also has a favorable impact on our cholesterol. Besides decreasing our total cholesterol, olive oil also lowers the bad (LDL) cholesterol and makes it less susceptible to oxidative damage by free radicals. The good (HDL) cholesterol is maintained or increased with olive oil consumption and the total cholesterol to HDL ratio is improved.

A Mediterranean diet with olive oil also helps with weight loss. A study in Boston revealed that a diet which included olive oil and nuts resulted in sustained weight loss over 18 months compared to a low fat diet. Compliance was also better, as the group on the Mediterranean diet did not feel like they were on a diet.

Whole grains

Whole grains, an integral part of the Mediterranean diet, are non-refined grains that provide us with energy and nutrition. In addition, whole grains help us decrease our risk of heart disease, diabetes and cancer. The whole grain kernel consists of an outer layer (bran), a middle layer (complex carbohydrates and protein) and an inner layer (vitamins, minerals and protein). The process of refining, common outside the Mediterranean region, destroys the outer and inner layer of the grain. This results in grains that lack fiber and disease fighting vitamins and phytochemicals. Examples of whole grains common to the Mediterranean diet are whole wheat, buckwheat, whole wheat pasta, brown rice, oatmeal, kasha, quinoa and whole barley.

Nuts

Nuts, like olive oil, have been an integral part of the Mediterranean diet since antiquity. Nut consumption lowers cholesterol and decreases the risk of coronary heart disease. Nuts such as almonds and walnuts are rich in monounsaturated fat and omega-3 fatty acids. They also are a good source of fiber and vitamin E. Nuts are an excellent snack that leads to satiety and weight loss. Regular nut consumption has been shown to lower the risk of heart disease.

Beans (Legumes)

Beans have significant health benefits and are consumed on a regular basis in the Mediterranean region. Beans are a rich source of soluble and insoluble fiber and they help reduce cholesterol. In addition, beans are an excellent source of protein and vitamins. Regular bean consumption lowers the risk of heart disease, cancer and diabetes. Finally, beans help to curb appetite due to their high fiber content.

Red wine

Moderate alcohol consumption lowers the risk of coronary heart disease. Red wine, often part of a Mediterranean meal, is felt to have several advantages over other forms of alcohol. Red wine contains polyphenols and resveratrol, two substances that help to promote heart health. Resveratrol, a powerful antioxidant, is more abundant in red wine than white wine. This compound lowers bad LDL cholesterol and raises good HDL cholesterol. It also has a beneficial impact on clotting. Remember, alcohol should be consumed in moderation. Wine consumption should not exceed one to two (4 oz.) glasses per day.

Grape juice — specifically purple grape juice – also lowers the risk of heart attack. The mechanism is felt to be similar to that of red wine. For those individuals who do not wish to consume wine, grape juice is an excellent alternative. Since most heart attacks occur in the morning, many patients with cardiovascular risk factors have a small glass of purple grape juice with breakfast.

Fresh fruit and vegetables

Go to any market in the Mediterranean basin and there will be a bountiful supply of fresh fruits and vegetables grown in that region. Vitamins, minerals, fiber and complex carbohydrates are contained in fruits and vegetables. Phytonutrients are nutrients concentrated in the skin of fruits and vegetables. These phytonutrients are powerful antioxidants and they help to improve our immune system. This leads to a decrease in heart disease and cancer. It is recommended that we eat a variety of food colors (oranges, blueberries, red apples, spinach, yellow squash, etc.) in order to get all the phytochemicals and nutritional benefits that fruits and vegetables provide.

Fish

Oily fish provide us with a rich source of protein and omega-3 fatty acids. Omega-3 fatty acids have a favorable impact on our cholesterol and triglyceride levels and reduce our risk for heart attack. They also help to reduce inflammation. Fatal cardiac arrhythmias with sudden death are decreased with consumption of omega-3 fatty acids. Examples of oily fish rich in omega-3 fatty acid content are salmon, albacore tuna, mackerel, sardines, herring and trout. Consumed in moderation, fish is beneficial to our heart health.

Fiber

Fiber is important in our diet since it lowers cholesterol as well as promotes proper gastrointestinal function and decreases the incidence of certain types of cancer. We should consume 25 to 30 grams of fiber a day. Unfortunately, most Americans consume less than ten grams of fiber per day. Oatmeal, high-fiber bread, whole grain cereals and beans are examples of food rich in their fiber content.

Water

It is essential that we consume an adequate amount of water each day. We should drink at least six to eight glasses or 48 ounces of water per day. If we don't consume enough water we become dehydrated. When we become dehydrated our serum viscosity rises, our blood becomes thick and does not flow smoothly and we are more likely to have a sudden thrombosis or clot. This can result in a sudden heart attack or stroke. The situation is aggravated by caffeine and alcohol consumption since both caffeine and alcohol have diuretic properties which further aggravates dehydration. People who live in tropical climates are even more at risk for dehydration since they have significant fluid loss through perspiration. Many feel that drinking water also helps to curb the appetite, thereby aiding those on a weight reduction diet.

Low fat dairy products

Low fat yogurt, soy milk, goat milk and low fat cheese provide a source of calcium which helps to build strong and healthy bones. Milk is consumed to a lesser degree in the Mediterranean region compared to milk consumption in a typical Western diet. Whole milk and butter milk are high in saturated fat and is generally avoided in the Mediterranean diet.

Daily exercise

Daily exercise is part of the Mediterranean lifestyle. Whether it's walking to the market or working on a farm, regular daily exercise is customary. Exercise raises our good cholesterol, lowers our blood pressure and decreases stress. Indeed, regular exercise has numerous health benefits which help us stay healthy and provides us with a sense of well-being.

Avoid stress

People living in Mediterranean countries tend to have less stress in their daily lives compared to their American counterparts. They spend more time enjoying their meals with family and friends. They often relax and take a nap after lunch. Smile, laugh and enjoy life — a prescription for a long and happy life.

What Is Wrong With the Popular Fad Diets?

Americans have always been enamored with "quick fix" diets which promise rapid and sustained weight loss. The problem with these diets is that they lack validity. There is no scientific basis or long-term data demonstrating the effectiveness of these diets for sustained weight loss or long-term health. I consider these diets to be fad diets!

Low carbohydrate diets, high in saturated fat and protein, are felt by many physicians to be suspect. There have been a number of articles in the scientific literature which have questioned the wisdom of recommending a diet high in saturated fat despite the concerns in the medical community linking saturated fat consumption with heart disease and cancer.

Strict vegetarian diets, on the other hand, are hard to follow and not palatable for most Americans.

Fad diets often promise quick and easy weight loss. The sad truth is that although some diets may result in early weight loss, the weight is quickly gained back and at the end of one year the decline in weight is similar from one diet to another.

- **Low fat diets (Ornish and Pritican):** Low fat and high carbohydrate diets (mainly vegetarian). These diets are hard to follow and not palatable for most Americans.
- **AHA (American Heart Association) Diet:** Low fat diet however HDL-cholesterol (good cholesterol) may decrease and heart disease can progress despite this diet. The Mediterranean diet contains more monounsaturated fat and omega-3 fat than

the AHA diet and is associated with a lowered risk of heart attack and cardiac death.

- **Low carbohydrate (Atkins and South Beach):** There is no long term data demonstrating clinical benefit. Concern about increasing the risk of heart disease and cancer make these diets suspect according to many doctors. High protein, low carbohydrate "ketogenic" diets often lead to quick early weight loss due to water loss. This diruesis (water loss) is due to depletion of muscle and liver glycogen (3 grams of water are lost for every 1 gram of glycogen). This process can lead to fluid and electrolyte changes that can potentially cause serious cardiac arrhythmias in a susceptible individual. It can also harm the kidneys and other vital organs. The impact of these diets on our cholesterol is unpredictable. Some people can have a significant rise in their bad LDL cholesterol as a result of the increase in saturated fat in these diets.

It is important to remember that a Mediterranean diet does not restrict carbohydrates. Low carbohydrate diets that achieve an "artificial" weight loss due to water loss from glycogen breakdown and ketosis are usually not effective in the long run. Rather, a Mediterranean diet is a proven dietary approach designed to promote long term health.

In summary, low carbohydrate diets are no more successful in the long run than well balanced diets with respect to weight loss. They are however potentially more dangerous than conventional diets leading many physicians in the scientific community to not recommend these diets. Some of the reported side effects and complications of low carb – high protein/fat diets include a potential increase risk of:

- Coronary heart disease
- Cancer
- Diabetes
- Kidney failure
- Kidney stones
- Cardiac arrhythmia (disorder of the heart rhythm)

- Elevated cholesterol
- Elevated CRP (a marker of inflammation)
- Deficiency of micronutrients
- Optic neuropathy
- Dehydration
- Gout
- Impaired cognitive function
- Halitosis (bad breath)

The Miami Mediterranean Diet differs from "low carb" diets in a number of ways:

- The Miami Mediterranean Diet is based on a traditional Mediterranean approach, therefore there is a significant reduction in saturated animal fat compared to "low carb" diets.
- The Miami Mediterranean Diet does not restrict healthy carbohydrates. Instead, fruits, vegetables and whole grains are encouraged throughout the diet.
- The Miami Mediterranean Diet advises portion control rather than an unlimited quantity of food with each meal.
- The Miami Mediterranean Diet recommends extra-virgin olive oil as the principal source of fat.
- The Miami Mediterranean Diet advises daily exercise and relaxation – remember, this is a lifestyle, not just a diet.

Forget fad diets! Follow the diet which is delicious and associated with long-term health – a Mediterranean diet! It is safe and effective and has been around for thousands of years.

Fat: The Good, The Bad and The Ugly

There are three types of fat in our diet: unsaturated fat, saturated fat and trans-fat.

- Unsaturated fats are good fats and include polyunsaturated fats and monounsaturated fats. Omega-3 and Omega 6 fatty acids are polyunsaturated fats. Oily fish, vegetables and nuts are examples of omega-3-fatty acids and are cardioprotective (decrease the risk of heart disease). Vegetable oils like soybean, sunflower and corn oils, are examples of omega-6 fatty acids and are neutral with regard to heart health. Nuts, seeds, and olive oil are examples of foods with cardioprotective monounsaturated fats. Monounsaturated fats are thought to be beneficial since they have a positive impact on our cholesterol ratio and they help to decrease inflammation.

- Saturated fats are bad fats since they raise the bad LDL-cholesterol and increase the risk of heart disease and cancer. Saturated fats are found in animal products, such as red meat, butter and lard as well as some oils, like coconut and palm oils.

- Then there are trans fatty acids or trans-fats. These fats are particularly harmful to our health since they raise the bad LDL-cholesterol and lower the good HDL-cholesterol. Trans-fat consumption is linked to heart disease, cancer, diabetes and obesity. In fact, certain countries have actually banned trans-fats from their food supply! Trans-fats are found in foods such as margarine, French fries, potato chips, cookies, crackers and baked goods. The problem with the American diet is that we consume too much saturated fat and trans-fat. Trans-fats are not naturally occurring. They're manufactured by taking oils, mainly vegetable oils, and putting them through a process called hydrogenation. Trans-fats were developed so that foods wouldn't become rancid and could last longer on the shelf. We can get an idea that a product contains trans-fat if partially or fully hydrogenated fat appears on the nutritional label.

The goal of a healthy diet is to limit consumption of saturated fats and trans-fats and follow the principles of a Mediterranean type diet with fresh fruits and vegetables, whole grains, monounsaturated fats, omega-3 fatty acids and fiber. Finally, avoid processed food and refined sugar, drink plenty of water and exercise daily.

Carbohydrates: Simple and Complex

Carbohydrates are a source of energy and nutrition that is essential to good health. Simple carbohydrates are sugars which are quickly absorbed into our bloodstream and provide an immediate source of energy. Examples of simple carbohydrates are candy and soda. Complex carbohydrates, also known as polysaccharides or starches, are made of long strands of simple sugars and are broken down and metabolized more slowly and provide the body with energy over a longer period of time. They are also more filling and help to curb the appetite. A previous study concluded that altering the diet in favor of more complex carbohydrates and less saturated fat may decrease the incidence of obesity. Whole wheat bread and pasta, potatoes, oatmeal and apples are examples of complex carbohydrates.

The glycemic response is the speed which a food is able to increase blood sugar or glucose. The glycemic index is a ranking of food based on their glycemic response. White bread is given a glycemic index of 100. Foods which increase blood sugar faster than white bread have a glycemic index greater than 100; foods which increase blood sugar slower than white bread are assigned a glycemic index less than 100.

A strategy for healthy eating is to select foods with a low glycemic index. This means selecting complex carbohydrates with more fiber and less sugar. This will improve blood glucose levels and decrease the likelihood of developing diabetes and heart disease. It will also lead to satiety and help to decrease weight gain leading to obesity.

Don't despair – you do not need to memorize the glycemic index of different foods. The Mediterranean diet is ideally suited for consuming healthy carbohydrates with a low glycemic index. Whole grains, nuts, fresh fruits and vegetables contain the "good carbohydrates" essential for a healthy diet. The "bad carbohydrates" which contain refined sugar and have a high glycemic index are not a part of a typical Mediterranean cuisine.

Clinical Vignette
S.D.

I've been a patient of Doctor Ozner's now for four years and I couldn't be happier. I'm feeling great and thanks to him I have not needed a repeat heart catheterization.

About four and one half years ago, I awoke early, about five A.M., with the most horrible pain in my chest and extreme shortness of breath. In a panic and an unbelievable sense of impending doom I woke my husband who immediately called 911. The rest is history. Through the grace of God and $40,000.00 dollars later I had survived a major heart attack. Seven months prior to this I had experienced a few minor symptoms that lead me to see a group of doctors who tested me, placed a stent in my coronary artery and said I could go home and relax, because they had taken care of my problem. Now that same group of doctors were telling me that I was stable following a second stent, nevertheless they told me to return to the emergency room if I experienced any more chest pain. I couldn't help feeling that I needed to do more than wait for the next event to occur. I personally needed to take steps that would help me avoid another such experience.

I am 52 years old, the mother of two grown children and the grandmother of three adorable grandkids. I desperately want to be around to enjoy them and to spend those coveted golden years with my husband. There had to be more that could be done for me besides leaving the hospital with a second stent and instructions to go immediately to the closest emergency room if I had more pain. I felt it was just a matter of time until I would once again find myself lying on an ER stretcher praying that my heart would continue to beat and give me a few more years. It seemed that the only thing between me and death was an element of luck. The word despondent barely depicted my anxiety.

I became determined to learn more about heart disease and what additional options where available to me. About three or four months later my husband heard of a cardiologist in Miami, Florida who exclusively practices cardiovascular prevention. We were told that he gives lectures to other physicians and healthcare providers as well as to the general public. After researching his name and credentials, I finally began to feel there was hope for me. We heard stories of how he believes in aggressive prevention with diet and exercise as well as medications to prevent future heart attacks. I therefore made an appointment to see him.

He started me on a regime of medical therapy to get my cholesterol, blood pressure and blood sugar to goal. He also started me on his prevention diet which is based on a Mediterranean approach. Both my husband and I now use this diet as well as my oldest daughter and her husband. It's now 2 1/2 years later and I feel great. I've lost a lot of weight and have maintained a normal weight since I started his diet regimen. At first when he mentioned lifestyle changes and diet, I panicked. I had previously tried other diets for weight control but after the initial weight loss I would eventually gain the weight back and then some. I had tried almost every diet. The results were the same, a seesaw pattern of weight loss then gain. I also questioned the logic of the low carb diets, since they allowed generous portions of red meat and other high fat foods. I have come to realize that most of these diets just don't make much sense, especially for long term health. Doctor Ozner explained how the Mediterranean diet has been in existence for thousands of years in the Mediterranean regions of the world and has been proven over the past 50 years to reduce the risk of heart disease. I've lost the weight by following the dietary guidelines. I have cut my portion size of food and started an exercise routine of daily walking. I've kept the excess weight off and have found that this is a diet I can live with for the rest of my life. As a matter of fact, it's a way of life that my entire family embraces. Thanks to Dr. Ozner, I have re-gained my health!

The Important Role of Antioxidant Vitamins and Micronutrients

Antioxidant vitamins and micronutrients are important for our health. The problem with the typical American diet is that we no longer consume fresh, non-processed, foods. The processing of foods unfortunately removes many of the vitamins, phytochemicals and micronutrients that we need for our long-term health. The vitamins that are found in fresh fruits and vegetables help to guard against the oxidation of our bad (LDL) cholesterol. Oxidized LDL cholesterol is more apt to cause clogged arteries. We also need micronutrients to protect us against the ravages of atherosclerosis and cancer. We need to keep the ratio of plant foods to animal foods at a high level. It is therefore abundantly clear that the Mediterranean diet, which emphasizes consumption of fresh fruits and vegetables, will ensure that we have proper nutrients and anti-oxidants which will help us fight disease.

What are Plant Sterols?

Plant sterols (phytosterols) are similar to cholesterol, an animal sterol. They are found in fruits, vegetables, nuts, seeds, cereals and legumes. They are also present in spreads such as Take Control and Smart Balance. Plant sterols are beneficial since they can interfere with the intestinal absorption of cholesterol, thereby lowering cholesterol levels. A Mediterranean diet provides an abundant amount of plant sterols.

The Thrifty Gene

The thrifty gene allows us to store food, in the form of fat, which is not immediately needed as an energy source. This has allowed us to survive as a species. In times of famine, when food was scarce, stored fat could be utilized as an energy source. Unfortunately, modern man has an abundant food supply and stored fat becomes detrimental to health.

Abdominal fat is more than just a cosmetic problem. These fat stores secrete inflammatory proteins which can lead to disease states such as heart disease, cancer and diabetes. The message is very clear. We should avoid obesity by consuming the proper amount of calories and engaging in regular exercise.

The Secret To Weight Loss

Simply stated, in order to achieve weight loss, one must burn more calories than one consumes. Americans consume too many calories! We tend to have several large meals and then begin snacking in the evening while we sit and watch TV. This endless cycle of excessive caloric intake combined with our sedentary lifestyle is the reason why obesity is a major public health threat. We must learn to eat smart. First we must understand that in order to eat smart we must limit the portions of food we eat. We must become a nation of calorie counters. Calories in minus calories out must be a negative number if we are to lose weight. There is no magical weight loss diet. Millions of dollars are spent each year on weight loss programs. Save your money! Instead, begin counting calories throughout the day. Next, know how many calories you burn when exercising. This simple program of knowing your calories in and calories out will take the guesswork out of dieting. Become a calorie counter! Become a calorie burner! You will lose weight.

How Does the Mediterranean Diet Achieve Weight Loss?

Is there a magical diet which results in sustained weight loss irrespective of the amount of calories consumed with food? The answer is no! Weight loss occurs when we burn more calories than we consume.

The Mediterranean diet is an ideal diet for weight loss. People who live in the Mediterranean region and follow a Mediterranean diet and lifestyle are leaner than their American counterparts who consume the typical Western diet. Food consumed in a typical Mediterranean diet can lead to weight loss in a number of ways:

- Consumption of food with a high fiber content leads to a feeling of being "full" (satiety). Fruit and vegetables, beans, nuts and whole grains are a rich source of fiber.
- Fat consumption in the Mediterranean diet also leads to satiety. Olive oil, nuts and fish are examples of Mediterranean food with a high (unsaturated) fat content.
- Complex carbohydrates are part of Mediterranean meals. Simple carbohydrates and refined sugar, linked with obesity are avoided.
- Trans - fats, associated with weight gain and obesity, are avoided in a Mediterranean diet. Non-processed food, such as fresh fruits and vegetables, are encouraged.
- Drinking an adequate amount of water (48 oz. or more) daily is advised. People often acknowledge that ample water consumption helps them curb their appetite.
- Food is not "super sized" in Mediterranean countries like it is in America. It is the quality of food, not the quantity of food! Eat sensible portions. The idea is to enjoy your meal in a relaxed manner with family and friends.

Exercise is also part of the Mediterranean lifestyle. Daily activity and exercise helps to burn calories. This leads to weight control and avoidance of obesity.

Therefore, if one wants to begin a diet that promotes nutrition and good health along with weight control then the Mediterranean diet is the answer! Remember that the Mediterranean diet is the only diet with long-term studies proving its health benefits. Forget fad diets! Isn't this is the type of diet that you would want for your family and yourself for a lifetime?

Is the Mediterranean Diet Palatable?

The Mediterranean diet is more than just palatable – it is delicious! Don't take my word for it – try it! The recipes contained in this book list foods that are easy to find in the grocery store, easy to prepare in the kitchen and taste great. Instead of processed foods, you will begin a diet of fresh fruits and vegetables, garlic, olive oil, whole grains, pasta, low fat yogurt and cheese, fish, chicken and lamb. You will quickly lose your addiction to fast foods, processed foods, refined sugar and foods high in saturated fat and trans-fat. You will be healthier, happier and leaner!

Clinical Vignette
J. H.

I have always been a quick fix weight loss junkie. I have jumped from one fad diet to another. It's not that I didn't take these diets seriously, I did. I tried protein shakes, miracle pills, starvation diets and even low carb diets. The Atkins and South Beach diets really sounded good to me because you could eat as much as you wanted, still have a few carbs and a variety of meat without having to worry about portion size and without having to exercise. WHAT COULD BE BETTER!

At first I lost 16 pounds. FABULOUS! The only trouble was that I always regained the weight. It was becoming a vicious cycle. Sadly I finally came to realize that these diets just didn't work.

But I knew I had to do something. You see, I'm a 38 year old Hispanic overweight male who otherwise is in good health. I have no symptoms but I have a strong family history of heart disease. My father had a heart attack early in life and died of a second heart attack at the age of 54. My aunt has a history of diabetes and my uncle had a stroke and subsequently died of a heart attack at the age of 61. My sister who is also overweight has recently been diagnosed with diabetes.

Because of this strong family history I saw Doctor Ozner a year ago. He started me on his Mediterranean prevention diet. I've been on it now for a little over a year and have successfully lost 28 pounds and have continued to actually keep the weight off. I have enjoyed this diet and found it quite easy to adhere to. I've not only lost weight but I have much more energy and feel healthier and physically stronger. I eat a wide variety of delicious healthy foods from every food group and I exercise daily (walking). This is a lifestyle change for me. I'm really pleased with the results I have seen and strongly recommend the Miami Mediterranean dietary guidelines. The best part is that this diet is delicious and it's easy to follow. With this change in lifestyle and diet, I feel that I will live a longer and healthier life.

Too Much Intervention – Not Enough Prevention

There are too many interventional cardiovascular procedures performed in this country on stable patients with coronary artery disease. Rather than relying on coronary artery bypass surgery and coronary stent placement for treatment, we should adopt an aggressive prevention approach so as to obviate the need for high-risk, expensive invasive procedures.

Needless to say, there are situations where surgical or cardiac catheterization procedures are not only needed but indeed may be lifesaving. This is especially true for unstable patients with impending or active heart attacks. However the vast majority of patients treated in the physician's office are not unstable. Rather, they are stable patients who either have risk factors for coronary heart disease or they actually have stable blockages in their arteries. A healthy lifestyle with proper diet, exercise and stress reduction, along with medications, if necessary, is our best defense against heart disease.

What is needed in this country is an aggressive prevention strategy - a strategy that will modify risk factors with lifestyle changes (diet, exercise, smoking cessation and stress management) and a strategy that will treat the genetic risk factors for coronary heart disease (cardiovascular medications). Aggressive prevention means more than just watching your diet and exercising on the weekends. Instead, an aggressive prevention approach means a radical change in an individual's lifestyle, as well as aggressive pharmacological treatment, if needed, to normalize risk factors for heart disease. An aggressive prevention approach results in lower cholesterol, plaque stabilization and can potentially eliminate the need for intervention, thereby avoiding high-risk surgical procedures. The optimal approach is to discuss all prevention and treatment strategies with your physician.

It is therefore beneficial to adopt a policy of aggressive cardiovascular prevention. Be proactive in your battle against heart disease and hopefully you will live a long, happy and heart - healthy life.

Stress: The Silent Killer

Stress is often the last modifiable risk factor to be discussed. This does not mean that stress is the least important risk factor — indeed it may be the most important! The problem with stress is that it cannot be measured like cholesterol or blood pressure. In addition, stress for one may not be stress for another.

Chronic stress increases stress hormones, such as cortisol and adrenaline. These stress hormones increase blood pressure, cause our heartbeat to become irregular and increase our likelihood of forming blood clots.

It is important to remember that it is not stress that kills you — it is distress or how one handles stress. I am reminded of two bullfighters from Barcelona. Pepe and Poncho were having lunch before the two matadors were to enter the stadium. Pepe said "Poncho isn't this great — I love bullfighting and I live to enter the stadium and fight the bull in front of all the people". Poncho replied "that's great Pepe but I hate what I do for a living — I have constant nightmares of being gored by the bull and my stomach is tied up in knots days before the bullfight". Here are two men in the same profession with completely opposite views regarding the stress of their occupation.

Studies have shown that chronic stress significantly increases the risk of heart attack. To make matters worse, those individuals who are "hot reactors" are especially prone to cardiovascular calamities. These are individuals who have a short fuse, are impatient and have a high hostility index. Often these individuals have no hobbies or activities which allow them to vent and blow off steam.

What then is the treatment for stress? First, let's be realistic — we all have periods of stress in our lives. Some unfortunately have more stress than others. Regardless, the first approach in handling stress is to take a realistic view of those factors which are responsible for stress in our lives and try our best to modify them. Next, I recommend a physical exercise program — not because exercise eliminates stress but rather people who exercise are better able to handle stress. There is a physiological explanation for the beneficial effects of exercise on stress. People who engage in regular aerobic exercise have lower catecholamine levels — in other words their adrenaline levels are lower and rise less dramatically with stressful situations.

In addition to a regular exercise program I encourage my patients to begin relaxation response training, yoga, self-hypnosis or meditation. Finally, prayer offers significant stress reduction for some individuals. If these lifestyle changes do not result in a significant reduction in stress then one should consider appropriate counseling with a psychologist or psychiatrist.

The Mediterranean diet and lifestyle can help reduce our level of stress. Meals are enjoyed with family and friends in a relaxed fashion with ample time for friendly conversation. Often a short nap or "siesta" follows the meal. Regular exercise is part of everyday life. It is no wonder that people following a Mediterranean diet and lifestyle have less stress and live longer and happier lives.

10 Steps For Stress Reduction

- Exercise daily
- Relax after meals
- Meditation
- Prayer
- Enjoy a close relationship with family and friends
- Set realistic goals in life
- Live within your means
- Yoga
- Enjoy hobbies & interests outside of your work
- Have a positive outlook in life and never lose your sense of

humor.
- Laugh, smile and enjoy life!

Exercise Daily — Your Heart Will Thank You

Physical inactivity with a sedentary lifestyle, along with poor dietary habits, has lead to the epidemic of obesity in America. Unfortunately we have become a nation of "couch potatoes". Getting people to exercise is difficult. We use the elevator instead of stairs. We ride in golf carts instead of walking. We park as close as possible in order to walk the fewest number of steps to the store. We must incorporate exercise into our daily activities.

Exercise does not necessarily mean jogging five miles a day. Simply walking for 30 minutes a day, 5 days a week has been shown to decrease the risk of heart attack and cardiovascular death. The cardiovascular benefits of regular aerobic exercise is significant. Besides decreasing the risk of heart attack, a regular exercise program will also reduce fatigue and stress, strengthen our bones and decrease the likelihood of osteoporosis and arthritis, improve our pulmonary function and generally provide us with a sense of well-being.

Obesity is closely affiliated with physical inactivity. Obesity in this country is epidemic. We consume more calories than we need and we do not burn calories with a proper exercise program. This is true not only in adults but also in children and adolescents. As a result of this alarming increase in obesity in the United States we now have a profound increase in diabetes. Those individuals who develop diabetes significantly increase their risk for the development of cardiovascular disease. Needless to say the solution should be education — education directed at getting people to eat properly and education to get people to begin an exercise program. Unfortunately we always look for the quick fix. The diet industry is a multibillion dollar business and yet the basic principle in achieving weight loss is simple: get the calories out (through physical activity and exercise) to exceed the calories in.

A Mediterranean lifestyle includes daily exercise. Walk at least 30 minutes per day. Daily exercise is as important to our health as a proper diet. Be heart smart – exercise daily and follow the dietary principles outlined in this book and you will reduce your risk of heart attack and stroke.

5 Simple & Easy Exercise Tips:
- Walk in place for 30 minutes while watching your favorite TV show – get off the couch!
- Park further away from your destination (office, store, etc) and enjoy a short walk
- Climb stairs instead of using the elevator
- Use a pedometer – strive for 10,000 steps per day
- Walk for the initial part of your lunch break – then eat lunch.

The Atherogenic Metabolic Stew: A Deadly Brew

If you ask most people "what is the cause of heart disease" their reply will be "cholesterol". Cholesterol may be good or bad. Good (HDL) cholesterol helps to remove bad (LDL) cholesterol from our arteries. Triglycerides represent another lipid or fat which can contribute to plaque buildup in our arteries.

There are however many other risk factors which can be measured with a blood test that increase our likelihood of developing heart disease. Besides cholesterol and triglycerides, numerous other risk factors have been identified:

- Homocysteine is a protein in the blood which has been linked to vascular damage and atherosclerosis.
- Fibrinogen is another protein which can lead to clotting if elevated.
- Infectious agents, such as viruses and bacteria, have also been implicated. Chlamydia pneumonia is an example of an infectious agent which some investigators have linked to atherosclerotic coronary heart disease and heart attack.
- Lipoprotein (a) is a "bad" cholesterol particle which increases the risk of heart attack and stroke.
- High sensitivity C reactive protein (hs – CRP) is a marker of inflammation which is linked to an increase risk of

cardiovascular disease.

- Pattern B trait is associated with small dense bad (LDL) cholesterol particles which increase the likelihood of atherosclerotic plaque buildup leading to heart disease and stroke.

Collectively all of the risk factors mentioned above as well as other emerging risk factors have been termed the atherogenic metabolic stew. The task of the preventive cardiologist is to treat all of the known risk factors thereby decreasing this deadly stew. This will result in a decrease in atherosclerotic plaque buildup as well as a decrease in the risk of heart attack, stroke and peripheral vascular disease.

Your First Symptom May Be Your Last

It would be nice if we had a warning system that alerted us that an impending heart attack would occur in the near future. With such a system in place we would simply wait until we developed a warning before we sought medical attention. Many people think that the presence of chest pain is our warning system. Unfortunately, in nearly two-thirds of men and one-half of women, the first symptom is sudden death or an acute myocardial infarction (heart attack).

We have to take action before we become symptomatic. In many respects atherosclerotic coronary heart disease acts like a silent killer — we are completely unaware of its presence in our body until a plaque ruptures and a cardiovascular catastrophe occurs. As physicians, if we wait until our patients become symptomatic with chest pain, then we have failed our patients. We must intervene with aggressive cardiovascular prevention prior to the onset of symptoms. This is the only strategy that will significantly decrease the risk of heart attack and death. We must aggressively attack the risk factors for heart disease with lifestyle changes (diet, exercise, stress management, smoking cessation) as well as appropriate medical therapy when required. This is the only way to defeat this formidable enemy, cardiovascular disease. We must attack when the enemy is most easily defeated — prior to the onset of symptoms!

The Diabetes Epidemic and How To Prevent It

There is an epidemic in this country — diabetes. Why is the incidence of diabetes increasing — especially in our young adult population? The answer is simple — the typical American eats too much and doesn't exercise. The reason why diabetes is a major concern is that the majority of diabetics die from cardiovascular disease.

The role of exercise in promoting cardiovascular health and avoiding diabetes has not been adequately emphasized in this country. The number of obese children, adolescents and adults are increasing at an alarming rate. We are a nation of couch potatoes. Children are no longer required to take physical education in school. In addition, the hard physical work that has been associated with many occupations has disappeared. We now go to school or sit in our office for eight hours a day and then come home and sit in front of the computer or TV for another four hours. Regular exercise is as foreign to most Americans as bullfighting.

We must change our attitude towards diet and exercise. Proper exercise does not necessarily mean excessive or strenuous exercise. A regular walking program for 30 minutes to an hour per day will result in significant benefit. Weight lifting utilizing light weights in a repetitive fashion is also beneficial. Women also benefit greatly from regular exercise. Women who engage in regular exercise decrease their risk of heart disease. In addition, they improve their bone density thereby decreasing the likelihood of osteoporosis.

Dietary factors have also contributed to the alarming increase in diabetes. We "super – size" our meals and consume too many calories. We eat processed food containing refined sugar and trans-fats. Suffice it to say that we must decrease our caloric intake and increase our caloric expenditure.

The message is clear — in order to avoid obesity and diabetes, Americans must adopt lifestyle changes that include regular exercise and a proper diet. It is only with this type of preventative approach that we will decrease the incidence of diabetes. By decreasing the incidence of diabetes we will decrease the epidemic of heart disease in this country.

The Important Medications for Cardiovascular Disease Prevention

Cardiovascular disease prevention begins with lifestyle modification. A proper diet and exercise program, along with stress management and smoking cessation form the foundation of our heart disease prevention guidelines. There are people who nevertheless develop heart disease even though they follow these guidelines. These individuals have a genetic basis for their heart disease and require medications along with a healthy lifestyle. There are numerous medications which are used in our treatment of cardiovascular disease. In this chapter some of the important medications which are used for cardiovascular disease prevention will be discussed.

- HMG-CoA reductase inhibitors, also known as the statins, reduce cholesterol levels by decreasing the production of cholesterol in the body. Clinical trials that have evaluated the impact of statins on heart disease prevention have demonstrated a significant lowering of heart attack risk and death from coronary heart disease.

- Niacin, fibrates, resins and cholesterol absorption inhibitors can also lower cholesterol and triglyceride levels.

- ACE inhibitors are medications which lower blood pressure and help stabilize the blood vessel wall. They have been shown to lower heart attack risk in patients with heart disease risk factors.

- Beta blockers decrease blood pressure and heart rate by blocking adrenaline. These drugs are especially useful in patients who have hypertension and cardiac arrhythmias. In addition, beta blockers have been shown to reduce the risk of sudden death in certain high-risk patients with cardiovascular disease.

- Aspirin has been shown to decrease the risk of heart attack and stroke by blocking the effects of platelets, cells which contribute to thrombus or clot formation. Low-dose aspirin appears to be as effective as high dose aspirin for cardiovascular protection. Unless there is a contraindication to aspirin therapy, most physicians advise that all patients at risk for cardiovascular disease should take aspirin on a regular basis.

- Fish oil supplements have been shown to benefit cardiovascular health. In a large Italian study, more than 10,000 men and women with preexisting heart disease were given fish oil or placebo. Those taking fish oil capsules had a 45% reduction in their risk of sudden cardiac death compared to placebo. Fish oil has also been shown to decrease triglyceride levels.

Many other medications are used in cardiovascular disease prevention. Calcium channel blockers and angiotensin receptor blockers are examples of blood pressure medications which are used to treat patients with cardiovascular disease. New medications are being developed to battle heart disease. For example, a more efficient good (HDL) cholesterol, developed through genetic engineering, has been shown to decrease plaque buildup in our arteries.

It is important that all patients be aware of the medications which are available to treat cardiovascular disease and it is equally important that they understand the potential side effects of these medications. There is no substitute for regular medical follow-up and discussion between the patient and his or her physician to decide which medications are best for each individual's cardiovascular health.

Clinical Vignette
R.S.

I am a 48 year old male Executive who often works a 60 hour week and plays occasional tennis whenever I can fit it into my hectic schedule. I'm divorced and tend to eat out a lot, often just grabbing 2 double cheeseburgers with bacon and super - sized fries at the nearest fast food restaurant. I also eat potato chips for snacks. I seldom see a doctor, except for an occasional bad cold. Other than being slightly overweight by 15 pounds, I consider myself to be in fairly good health. When I was a young boy my parents always encouraged me to eat foods high in protein and fat because they thought those foods would make me strong and healthy. Except for the vegetables on my pizzas and fruit in my ice cream, I seldom consume fresh fruits or vegetables. Also, fish is just not part of my vocabulary.

One Sunday afternoon, about 6 months ago, I was playing a grueling game of tennis, when I suddenly developed tightness in my chest. It was severe enough to cause me to stop and take notice. Two days later I saw a doctor, which led me to a heart evaluation by a cardiologist and a subsequent heart catheterization with a stent placement in one of my major coronary arteries.

While I was hospitalized, I heard about Doctor Ozner from the nurses taking care of me. He had just given a lecture on heart disease prevention and they were discussing his prevention approach. It was then that I decided to make an appointment to see him.

He educated me about cardiovascular health and the role that diet, exercise and stress management play in maintaining good health. He said that I could significantly reduce the likelihood of having a heart attack if I changed my current lifestyle and eating habits. He gave me a book to read on heart disease prevention and literature on his Mediterranean prevention diet. After reviewing all the literature it became clear to me that a diet of high protein and saturated fat actually contributed to my chances of dying from a heart attack. I wanted a common sense approach. After trying the Miami Mediterranean diet, I realized it was not only a healthy and nutritious way to eat, but the food was also delicious! Although I still take medications, I have improved my diet and I exercise on a regular basis. I am confident that these measures will decrease my chances of having a heart attack or dying prematurely from heart disease.

What Is The Solution? It's Your Choice!

There are two different pathways that you can travel in the war against cardiovascular disease. The first pathway is called the dead end road. Those who travel down the dead end road refuse to learn about cardiovascular disease prevention. Their attitude is "I'll wait until I have chest pain and then I'll worry about it". They frequently criticize people who take medications and they say "medications have adverse side effects which can cause serious problems and I simply won't take them". They refuse to exercise or watch their diet. The dead end road eventually leads to the number one cause of death in the United States — cardiovascular disease.

The second pathway is called progress road. People who travel down progress road refuse to succumb to cardiovascular disease without a fight. They understand the basic principles of cardiovascular disease prevention. They maintain a heart healthy diet and exercise on a regular basis. They have appropriate blood tests to screen for cardiovascular disease and they understand the current guidelines for cholesterol and triglyceride management. If they have an elevated cholesterol or triglyceride level they seek out appropriate medical attention so they can receive proper treatment. Those who travel down the progress road have a much lower likelihood of being hospitalized with a heart attack or undergoing expensive cardiac catheterization and angioplasty. They are also much less likely to undergo coronary artery bypass surgery. Progress road ultimately leads to cardiovascular health!

Let us not underestimate our enemy — cardiovascular disease. It claims more lives than any other disease — every 30 seconds someone will die from a heart attack in this country. Certainly if we were fighting an enemy this formidable we would do whatever it takes to win the war. I hope that this book will provide you with the knowledge and motivation to take charge of your own cardiovascular well-being. Aggressive prevention should be your battle-cry and hopefully you will live a long, happy and heart healthy life.

PART TWO

A 14 Day Menu Plan

The Miami Mediterranean Diet is not a quick weight loss diet plan but rather a healthy nutritional plan that will help you reach and maintain your optimal weight. You may substitute any Mediterranean recipe for those listed in the 14 Day menu plan. In addition, you are encouraged to eat a variety of fresh fruits and vegetables (use olive oil or vegetable spread to flavor vegetables as desired). The recipes in this book are made from a variety of fresh, healthy, non-processed foods. The fat content listed in these recipes is mainly unsaturated fat (especially monounsaturated fat and omega-3 fat) with limited saturated fat and no appreciable trans-fat. Remember to exercise daily and adjust portion size to achieve ideal body weight. Bon appetit!

DAY 1

Breakfast

4 oz. glass of vegetable or fruit juice
1 slice whole wheat toast with extra-virgin olive oil or 1 teaspoon vegetable spread (such as Smart Balance or Benecol)
1 teaspoon jam
1/2 cup plain low-fat yogurt (sweetened with Splenda if desired) and 1/2 cup blueberries or strawberries
8 oz. water
Coffee or tea (soy or non-fat coffee creamer and Splenda, if desired)

Approx: 239 calories

Optional mid- morning snack:
10-20 almonds or walnuts
8 oz. water or non-caloric beverage

Lunch

Chickpea pita pocket (page 218)
1 medium apple, sliced and drizzled with honey
8 oz. water or non-caloric beverage

Approx: 319 calories

Optional mid-day snack:
10-20 almonds or walnuts
8 oz. water or non-caloric beverage

Dinner

1 jumbo clove roasted garlic, (page 253)
1/2 (6-inch) whole wheat pita loaf, split open and sprayed with olive
oil and herb seasonings of choice and toasted in the microwave or oven
until crispy
Goat cheese stuffed tomato salad (page 69)
Whole wheat linguine and mixed seafood (page 165)
Fresh vegetable of choice (flavor with olive oil or vegetable spread as
desired)
Drunken apricots (page 245)
8 oz. water
1 or 2 (4 oz.) glasses of red wine (or purple grape juice)
Coffee or tea (soy or non-fat coffee creamer and Splenda, if desired)

Approx: 761 calories

Optional evening snack:

1 apple or orange
8 oz. water

DAY 2

Breakfast

4 oz. glass of vegetable or fruit juice
1/2 cup dry oatmeal, cooked and sweetened with Splenda if desired
1 tablespoon dark seedless raisins
1 medium orange, sliced
8 oz. water
Coffee or tea (soy or non-fat coffee creamer and Splenda if desired)

Approx: 292 calories

Optional mid-morning snack:

10-20 almonds or walnuts
8 oz. water or non-caloric beverage

Lunch

Greek olive and feta cheese pasta salad (page 68)
1/2 (6-inch) whole wheat pita loaf, toasted if desired
1/8-inch fresh cantaloupe
8 oz. water or non-caloric beverage

Approx: 354 calories

Optional mid-day snack:

1 apple
8 oz. water or a non-caloric beverage

Dinner

Mediterranean mixed greens (page 74)
1 slice whole grain crusty bread with olive oil (extra-virgin)
1 slice of soft goat cheese
1 jumbo clove roasted garlic (page 253)
Italian poached scallops (page 159)
1/2 cup cooked wild rice
Strawberries in balsamic syrup (page 243)
8 oz. water
1 or 2 (4 oz.) glasses of red wine (or purple grape juice)
Coffee or tea (soy or non-fat coffee creamer and Splenda if desired)

Approx: 671 calories

Optional evening snack:

1 apple or orange
8 oz. water

DAY 3

Breakfast

1 oz. glass of vegetable or fruit juice
1/2 cup egg whites with diced onions, tomato and green peppers
1 slice whole wheat toast with olive oil (extra-virgin) or 1 teaspoon
vegetable spread (such as Smart Balance or Benecol)
1 teaspoon fruit jam
1 medium fresh peach or 1 large plum
8 oz. water
Coffee or tea (soy or non-fat coffee creamer and Splenda if desired)

Approx: 230 calories

Optional mid-morning snack:
10-20 almonds or walnuts
8 oz. water or non-caloric beverage

Lunch

Italian Minestrone soup with pesto (page 93)
1 slice whole grain crusty bread with olive oil (extra-virgin)
1/2 cup fresh raspberries
1/2 cup plain low-fat yogurt, sweetened with Splenda if desired
8 oz. water or non-caloric beverage

Approx: 390 calories

Optional mid-day snack:

1 apple
8 oz. water or a non-caloric beverage

Dinner

Simple Spanish salad (page 86)
1 jumbo clove roasted garlic (page 253)
1/2 (6-inch) whole wheat pita loaf, split open and sprayed with olive oil
and herb seasonings of choice and toasted until crispy in the oven or
microwave
1 slice soft goat cheese
6-8 marinated mixed olives (page 250)
Fresh vegetable of choice (flavor with olive oil or vegetable spread as
desired)
Chicken Piccata (page 176)
Honeydew sorbet (page 243)
8 oz. water
1 or 2 (4 oz.) glasses of red wine (or purple grape juice)
Coffee or tea (soy or non-fat coffee creamer and Splenda if desired)

Approx: 725 calories

Optional evening snack:

1 apple or orange
8 oz. water

DAY 4

Breakfast

4 oz. glass of vegetable or fruit juice
2 slices whole wheat toast
2 tablespoons fresh chunky peanut butter
2 teaspoons honey
1/2 ruby red grapefruit, Splenda if desired
8 oz. water
Coffee or tea (soy or non-fat coffee creamer and Splenda if desired)

Approx: 385 calories

Optional mid-morning snack:

10-20 almonds or walnut
8 oz. water or non-caloric beverage

Lunch

Light Caesar salad (page 81)
1 slice Marghertta pizza (page 109)
10-20 seedless grapes
8 oz. water or non-caloric beverage

Approx: 302 calories

Optional mid-day snack:

1 apple
8 oz. water or a non-caloric beverage

Dinner

1 clove of jumbo roasted garlic (page 253)
1/2 (6-inch) whole wheat pita loaf, sprayed with olive oil and herb seasonings of choice, toasted until crispy in the oven or microwave
Chilly tomato soup (page 98)
Fennel salad (page 77)
Fresh vegetable of choice (flavor with olive oil or vegetable spread as desired)
Spicy garlicky whole wheat capellini (page 151)
8 oz .water
Sweet plum compote (page 235)
1 or 2 (4 oz.) glasses of red wine (or purple grape juice)
Coffee or tea (soy or non-fat coffee creamer and Splenda if desired)

Approx: 786 calories

Optional evening snack:
1 apple or orange
8 oz. water

DAY 5

Breakfast

4 oz. glass of vegetable or fruit juice
1 slice whole wheat toast with olive oil (extra-virgin) or 1 teaspoon vegetable spread (such as Smart Balance or Benecol)
1 teaspoon fruit jam
1/2 cup plain low-fat yogurt, sweetened with Splenda if desired
1/2 cup blueberries or strawberries
8 oz. water
Coffee or tea (soy or non-fat coffee creamer and Splenda if desired)

Approx: 289 calories

Optional mid-morning snack:
10-20 almonds or walnuts
8 oz. water or non-caloric beverage

Lunch

Hearty bean soup (page 100)
1 slice whole grain bread with olive oil (extra-virgin) or 1 teaspoon vegetable spread (such as Smart Balance or Benecol)
3 fresh apricots
8 oz. water or non-caloric beverage

Approx: 414 calories

Optional mid-day snack:
1 apple
water or a non-caloric beverage

Dinner

4 tablespoons hummus
1/2 (6-inch) whole wheat pita loaf, split open, sprayed with olive oil and
herb seasonings of choice, toasted until crispy in the oven or microwave
4 tomato wedges topped with slivers of red onion, fresh grated
mozzarella cheese topped with chopped cilantro, drizzled with
1 teaspoon balsamic vinegar mixed with 1 teaspoon extra-virgin olive oil
Skewered Mediterranean grilled lamb and vegetables (page 134)
1/2 cup garlic rice (page 186)
Peach Marsala compote (page 234)
1 or 2 (4 oz.) glasses of red wine (or purple grape juice)
8 oz. water
Coffee or tea (soy or non fat coffee creamer and Splenda if desired)

Approx: 912 calories

Optional evening snack:
1 apple or orange
8 oz. water

DAY 6

Breakfast

4 oz. glass of vegetable or fruit juice
1/2 cup dry oatmeal, cooked and sweetened with Splenda if desired
1 tablespoon seedless black raisins
1 medium orange, sliced
8 oz. water
Coffee or tea (soy or non fat coffee creamer and Splenda if desired)

Approx: 292 calories

Optional mid-morning snack:
10-20 almonds or walnuts
8 oz. water or non-caloric beverage

Lunch

Veggie wrap (page 215)
Roasted peppers (page 182)
6-8 marinated mixed olives (page 250)
1 medium fresh pear
8 oz. water or non-caloric beverage

Approx: 601 calories

Optional mid-day snack:
1 apple
8 oz. water or non-caloric beverage

Dinner

1 jumbo clove roasted garlic (page 253)
1/2 (6-inch) whole wheat pita loaf, split open and sprayed with olive oil and herb seasonings, toasted until crispy in the oven or microwave
Mediterranean mixed greens (page 74)
Baked Tilapia (page 162)
Classic spinach and pine nuts (page 183)
Strawberries amaretto (page 246)
8 oz. water
1 or 2 (4 oz.) glasses of red wine (or purple grape juice)
Coffee or tea (soy or non-fat coffee creamer and Splenda if desired)

Approx: 597 calories

Optional evening snack:

1 apple or orange
8 oz. water

DAY 7

Breakfast

4 oz. glass of vegetable or fruit juice
1/2 cup egg whites with diced red onion, tomato and green peppers cooked into an omelet
1 slice of whole wheat toast with olive oil (extra-virgin) or 1 teaspoon vegetable spread (such as Smart Balance or Benecol)
1 teaspoon fruit jam
1 purple plum
8 oz. water
Coffee or tea (soy or non-fat coffee creamer and Splenda if desired)

Approx: 230 calories

Optional mid-morning snack:

10-20 almonds or walnuts
8 oz. water or non-caloric beverage

Lunch

Eggplant soup (page 106)
1 slice whole grain crusty bread - drizzled with extra-virgin olive oil and herb seasonings of choice
1 large kiwi fruit, sliced
1/2 cup fresh strawberries, sliced
8 oz. water or non-caloric beverage

Approx: 420 calories

Optional mid-day snack:

1 apple
8 oz. water or non-caloric beverage

Dinner

1 slice whole grain bread with extra-virgin olive oil and herb seasonings
of choice
6-8 marinated assorted olives (page 250)
Broccoli and fresh garlic (page 188)
Fettuccine with sun-dried tomatoes and goat cheese (page 173)
Fresh fruit kababs and cinnamon honey dip (page 238)
8 oz .water
1 or 2 (4 oz.) glasses of red wine (or purple grape juice)
Coffee or tea (soy or non-fat coffee creamer and Splenda if desired)

Approx: 1050 calories

Optional evening snack:

1 apple or orange
8 oz. water

DAY 8

Breakfast

1 oz. glass of vegetable or fruit juice
1/2 cup dry oatmeal, cooked and sweetened with Splenda if desired
1 tablespoon seedless dark raisins
1 small banana, sliced
8 oz. water
Coffee or tea (soy or non-fat coffee creamer and Splenda if desired)

Approx: 323 calories

Optional mid-morning snack:
10-20 almonds or walnuts
8 oz. water or non-caloric beverage

Lunch

Easy couscous parsley salad (page 87)
1/2 (6-inch) whole wheat pita loaf, toasted
Fresh fruit in yogurt
8 oz. water or non-caloric beverage

Approx: 331 calories

Optional mid-day snack:
1 apple
8 oz. water or non-caloric beverage

Dinner

1 jumbo clove roasted garlic (page 253)
1/2 (6-inch) whole wheat pita loaf, split open and sprayed with olive oil and herb seasonings of choice, toasted until crispy in the oven or microwave
Avocado salad (page 89)
Whole wheat spaghetti with anchovy and garlic sauce (page 172)
1/2-inch slice of honeydew or cantaloupe
8 oz. water
1 or 2 (4 oz.) glasses of red wine (or purple grape juice)
Coffee or tea (soy or non-fat coffee creamer and Splenda if desired)

Approx: 832 calories

Optional evening snack:

1 apple or orange
8 oz. water

DAY 9

Breakfast

4 oz. glass vegetable or fruit juice
2 slices whole wheat toast
2 tablespoons of fresh chunky peanut butter
2 teaspoons honey
1/2 ruby red grapefruit, Splenda if desired
8 oz. glass of water
Coffee or tea (soy or non-fat coffee creamer and Splenda if desired)

Approx: 385 calories

Optional mid-morning snack:
10-20 almonds or walnuts
8 oz. water or non-caloric beverage

Lunch

Chicken escarole soup (page 104)
1 slice whole grain crusty bread
1/8 wedge honeydew
8 oz. water or non-caloric beverage

Approx: 259 calories

Optional mid-day snack:
1 apple
8 oz. water or a non-caloric beverage

Dinner

2 stuffed grape leaves with lemon slices (page 248)
1/2 (6-inch) whole wheat pita loaf, split open and sprayed with olive oil and herb seasonings of choice, toasted until crispy in the oven or microwave
6-8 marinated assorted olives (page 250)
Baked eggplant with garlic and basil (page 205)
Steamed Seabass (page 154)
Cantaloupe sorbet (page 242)
8 oz. water
1 or 2 (4 oz.) glasses of red wine (or purple grape juice)
Coffee or tea (soy or non-fat coffee creamer and Splenda if desired)

Approx: 662 calories

Optional evening snack:
1 apple or orange
8 oz. water

DAY 10

Breakfast

4 oz. glass of vegetable or fruit juice
1 slice whole wheat toast with olive oil (extra-virgin) or 1 teaspoon vegetable spread (such as Smart Balance or Benecol)
1 teaspoon fruit jam
1/2 cup plain low-fat yogurt, sweetened with Splenda if desired
1/2 cup fresh blueberries or strawberries
8 oz. water
Coffee or tea (soy or non-fat coffee creamer and Splenda if desired)

Approx: 289 calories

Optional mid-morning snack:
10-20 almonds or walnuts
8 oz. water or non-caloric beverage

Lunch

Chilled stuffed pasta shells (page 184)
10-20 seedless grapes
1 large fresh tangerine
8 oz. water or non-caloric beverage

Approx: 292 calories

Optional mid-day snack:
1 apple
8 oz. water or non-caloric beverage

Dinner

1 jumbo clove roasted garlic (page 253)
1/2 (6-inch) whole wheat pita loaf, split open and sprayed with extra-virgin olive oil and herb seasonings of choice, toasted until crispy in the oven or microwave
Roasted red peppers (page 182)
Spicy shrimp with angel hair pasta (page 147)
Creme de Banana baked apples (page 241)
8 oz. water
1 or 2 (4 oz.) glasses of red wine (or purple grape juice)
Coffee or tea (soy or non-fat coffee creamer and Splenda if desired)

Approx: 735 calories

Optional evening snack:
1 apple or orange
8 oz. water

DAY 11

Breakfast

4 oz. glass of vegetable or fruit juice
1/2 cup dry oatmeal, cooked and sweetened with Splenda if desired
1 tablespoon seedless dark raisins
1 medium orange, sliced
8 oz. water
Coffee or tea (soy or a non-fat coffee creamer and Splenda if desired)

Approx: 292 calories

Optional mid-morning snack:

10-20 almonds or walnuts
8 oz. water or non-caloric beverage

Lunch

Garlicky cannellini beans (page 208)
1/2 (6-inch) whole wheat pita loaf, split open and sprayed with extra-virgin olive oil and seasonings of choice, toasted in the oven or microwave
1 medium apple sliced and drizzled with 1 teaspoon honey
8 oz. water or non-caloric beverage

Approx: 389 calories

Optional mid-day snack:

10-20 almonds or walnuts

8 oz. water or a non-caloric beverage

Dinner

Light Caesar salad (page 81)

1 slice whole grain bread, toasted

1 tablespoon extra-virgin olive oil with herb seasonings of choice

Lemon garlic asparagus (page 193)

Shrimp in spicy black bean sauce (page 178)

Garlic rice (page 186)

Strawberry and poached pears (page 229)

8 oz. water

1 or 2 (4 oz.) glasses of red wine (or purple grape juice)

Coffee or tea (soy or a non-fat coffee creamer and Splenda if desired)

Approx: 853 calories

Optional evening snack:

1 apple or orange

8 oz. water

DAY 12

Breakfast

4 oz. glass of vegetable or fruit juice
1/2 cup egg whites with diced onions, tomato and green peppers cooked into an omelet
1 slice whole wheat toast with extra-virgin olive oil or 1 teaspoon of a vegetable spread (such as Smart Balance or Benecol)
1 teaspoon fruit jam
1/2 small banana
8 oz .water
Coffee or tea (soy or non-fat coffee creamer and Splenda if desired)

Approx: 230 calories

Optional mid-morning snack:
10-20 almonds or walnuts
8 oz. water or non-caloric beverage

Lunch

Smoked fish and roasted pepper sandwich (page 221)
1/2 cup fresh raspberries
1/2 cup low-fat plain yogurt, Splenda if desired
8 oz. water or non-caloric beverage

Approx: 322 calories

Optional mid-day snack:
1 apple
8 oz. water or a non-caloric beverage

Dinner

Mediterranean mixed greens (page 74)
Tomato and fresh Parmesan cheese bruschette topping (page 252)
1 slice of crusty toasted French bread with extra-virgin olive oil
Fresh vegetable of choice (flavor with olive oil or vegetable spread as desired)
Bow tie pasta with eggplant and black olives (page 169)
Sweet Italian rice pudding (page 240)
8 oz. water
1 or 2 (4 oz.) glasses of red wine (or purple grape juice)
Coffee or tea (soy or non-fat coffee creamer and Splenda)

Approx: 984 calories

Optional evening snack:
1 apple or orange
8 oz. water

DAY 13

Breakfast

4 oz. glass of vegetable or fruit juice
2 slices whole wheat toast
2 tablespoons fresh chunky peanut butter
2 teaspoons honey
1/2 ruby red grapefruit, Splenda if desired
8 oz. water
Coffee or tea (soy or non-fat coffee creamer and Splenda if desired)

Approx: 385 calories

Optional mid-morning snack:
10-20 almonds or walnuts
8 oz. water or non-caloric beverage

Lunch

Chickpeas and garden vegetables (page 72)
1/2 (6-inch) whole wheat pita loaf, split open and sprayed with olive oil
and herb seasonings of choice toasted in the oven or microwave
1 medium orange, sliced
8 oz. water or non-caloric beverage

Approx: 325 calories

Optional mid-day snack:

1 apple

8 oz. water or a non-caloric beverage

Dinner

1 jumbo clove roasted garlic (page 253)

1/2 (6-inch) whole wheat pita loaf, split open and sprayed with olive oil and herb seasonings of choice, toasted until crispy in the oven or microwave

6-8 marinated assorted olives (page 250)

Grilled citrus salmon with garlic greens (page 140)

Grilled eggplant (page 210)

Strawberries and balsamic syrup (page 243)

8 oz. water

1 or 2 (4 oz.) glasses of red wine (or purple grape juice)

Coffee or tea (soy or a non-fat coffee creamer and Splenda if desired)

Approx: 653 calories

Optional evening snack:

1 apple or orange

8 oz. water

DAY 14

Breakfast

4 oz. glass vegetable or fruit juice
1/2 cup dry oatmeal, cooked and sweetened with Splenda if desired
1 tablespoon seedless dark raisins
1 medium orange, sliced
8 oz. water
Coffee or tea (soy or non-fat coffee creamer and Splenda if desired)

Approx: 292 calories

Optional mid-morning snack:
10-20 almonds or walnuts
8 oz. water or non-caloric beverage

Lunch

Spicy mushroom wrap (page 219)
1 medium fresh peach
8 oz. water or non-caloric beverage

Approx: 544 calories

Optional mid-day snack:
1 apple
8 oz. water or a non-caloric beverage

Dinner

1 jumbo clove roasted garlic (page 253)
1/2 (6-inch) whole wheat pita loaf, split open and sprayed with olive oil and herb seasonings of choice, toasted until crispy in the oven or microwave
Goat cheese stuffed tomato (page 69)
Fresh vegetable of choice (flavor with olive oil or vegetable spread as desired)
Pasta with red clam sauce (page 170)
Drunken peaches (page 244)
8 oz. water
1 or 2 (4 oz.) glasses of red wine (or purple grape juice)
Coffee or tea (soy or a non-fat coffee creamer and Splenda)

Approx: 830 calories

Optional evening snack:
1 apple or orange
8 oz. water

RECIPES

SALADS

GREEK OLIVE AND FETA CHEESE PASTA

Ingredients: Makes 4 servings

3 oz. of crumbled feta cheese
10 small Greek olives, pitted and coarsely chopped
1/4 cup fresh basil leaves, coarsely chopped
2 cloves garlic, finely minced
1 tablespoon extra-virgin olive oil
1/4 teaspoon finely chopped hot pepper
4 1/2 oz. Ziti pasta, cooked more or less al dente, drained and rinsed
1/2 red bell pepper, diced
1/2 yellow bell pepper, diced
2 plum tomatoes, seeded and diced

In a large serving bowl combine feta cheese, olives, basil, garlic, olive oil and hot peppers, set aside for 30 minutes. Add cooked pasta, red and yellow bell peppers and tomato, toss ingredients well. Cover and refrigerate for at least 1 hour, until well chilled. Toss again before serving. This salad goes well as a side dish to grilled lamb or fish.

Approx. 235 calories per serving
7g protein, 10g fat, 27g carbohydrates,
18mg cholesterol, 398mg sodium, 2g fiber

GOAT CHEESE STUFFED TOMATOES

Ingredients: Make 2 servings

2 medium ripe tomatoes
6-8 leaves arugula
3 oz. crumbled feta cheese
Salt and pepper to taste
Balsamic vinegar
Extra-virgin olive oil
Red onion, very thinly sliced
Fresh chopped parsley

Place 3-4 Arugula leaves around edges of salad plate. Cut tops (about 1/4-inch) off tomatoes. With a pairing knife, core out the center of the tomatoes, about 1/2-inch deep. Fill center and tops of tomatoes with crumbled feta cheese, add salt and pepper to taste. Drizzle stuffed tomatoes with balsamic vinegar and extra-virgin olive oil. Garnish with red onion slices and chopped parsley. Serve at room temperature.

> *Approx. 142 calories per serving*
> *7g protein, 13g fat, 7g carbohydrates,*
> *37mg cholesterol, 485mg sodium, 1g fiber*

CLASSIC TABBOULEH
(goes well with toasted herb seasoned whole wheat pita triangles)

Ingredients: Makes 4-6 servings as dinner salad or 8-10 as appetizer

3/4 cup bulgur
1 1/2 cups of water
2 cups freshly chopped parsley
3/4 cup chopped scallions, white and green parts
1/2 red bell pepper, diced
1/2 green pepper, diced
1/2 cup fresh mint, finely chopped
1/2 cup fresh lemon juice
1/2 cup extra-virgin olive oil
Sea salt and freshly ground pepper to taste
3 ripe plum tomatoes, peeled, seeded and diced
1 large cucumber, peeled, seeded and diced

In a small saucepan soak bulgur in water for 30 minutes. Drain bulgur through a sieve and allow it to dry thoroughly. Clean parsley under cold running water and press gently between paper towels to dry. Place bulgur, parsley, scallions, peppers and mint in a large bowl. Stir to mix well. In a separate bowl, whisk together lemon juice and oil. Season bulgur mixture with salt and pepper. Add lemon mixture to bulgur and toss. Add only enough lemon mixture to make salad moist but not runny. Fold in tomatoes and cucumbers. Cover and chill. Serve on a bed of greens, with seasoned pita wedges for dipping.

> **Approx. 177 calories per serving**
> **3g protein, 21g fat, 19g carbohydrates,**
> **0 cholesterol, 23mg sodium, 4g fiber**

SAVORY GREEK WHITE FAVA BEAN SALAD

Ingredients: Makes 4 servings

1 1/4 cups of dried white Fava beans- soak the beans over night in fresh water. (Water must cover the beans by twice its volume) In the morning drain beans and rinse with fresh water and drain well.
2-3 fresh sage leaves
Salt to taste
2 cloves garlic, finely minced
1 small onion, finely chopped
1 celery stalk, finely chopped
3 tablespoons of fresh lemon juice
1/2 teaspoon dried oregano
3 tablespoons extra-virgin olive oil
4 1/2 tablespoons of red wine vinegar
Freshly ground black pepper to taste

Combine pre-soaked drained beans and 1 quart of fresh water in a large pot bring to a boil. Add sage, cover pot and cook for about 45 minutes. Gently stir and add salt to taste and continue cooking for about another 15 minutes until beans are soft but not mushy. Remove from heat and drain. Let beans cool slightly then toss with garlic, onions, celery, lemon juice, oregano, oil and vinegar. Add freshly ground pepper to taste and chill for one hour or more before serving.

> *Approx. 253 calories per serving*
> *12g protein, 11g fat, 28g carbohydrates,*
> *0 cholesterol, 15mg sodium, 12g fiber*

CHICKPEAS AND GARDEN VEGETABLES

Ingredients: Makes 4 servings

2 tablespoons of freshly squeezed lemon juice
2 cloves of garlic, finely minced
1 tablespoon of fresh basil leaf, snipped
1/8 teaspoon freshly ground black pepper
1 (15 oz.) can of chickpeas, rinsed and well drained
2 cups coarsely chopped fresh broccoli
1/2 cup sliced fresh carrots
1 (7 1/2 oz.) can of diced tomatoes, do not drain
1 cup of cubed part-skim mozzarella cheese

In a large serving bowl combine lemon juice, garlic, basil, and ground pepper. Stir in beans, broccoli, carrots, tomatoes with juice, and cheese. Toss ingredients mixing well. Cover and refrigerate for at least 4 hours.

> **Approx. 195 calories per serving**
> **16g protein, 7g fat, 24g carbohydrates,**
> **17mg cholesterol, 411mg sodium, 2g fiber**

TANGY ORANGE ROASTED ASPARAGUS SALAD

Ingredients: Makes 6 servings

1 lb. fresh asparagus, trimmed and cut into 1/2 inch diagonal pieces
4 tablespoons of extra-virgin olive oil
Salt to taste
4 tablespoons of fresh sweet no pulp orange juice
1 tablespoon freshly squeezed lime juice
2 cloves finely minced garlic
Freshly ground black pepper to taste
7 cups of chopped fresh romaine lettuce
3 tablespoons toasted pine nuts
1 tablespoon of minced fresh basil leaf
Freshly grated Romano cheese (optional)

Preheat oven to 450 degrees F. Toss asparagus with 2 tablespoons of olive oil and salt to taste. Arrange asparagus in a baking dish in a single layer and place in oven. Roast until tender crispy, about 10 minutes. Set aside. In a bowl briskly whisk orange juice, lime juice, garlic and 2 tablespoons of olive oil, salt and pepper to taste. When ready to serve divide lettuce into 6 serving and arrange on salad plates and top with asparagus. Briefly whisk the dressing and pour over lettuce and asparagus salad. Top with toasted pine nuts and fresh minced basil. Garnish with a small amount of grated cheese if desired.

To toast pine nuts in the oven: Preheat oven to 375 degrees F. Place the nuts in one layer on a nonstick baking sheet. Bake at 450 degrees, stirring occasionally, until lightly browned. Remove from oven and allow too cool.

Approx. 124 calories per serving
4g protein, 10g fat, 6g carbohydrates,
0 cholesterol, 16mg sodium, 3g fiber

MEDITERRANEAN MIXED GREENS

Ingredients: Makes 4-6 servings

6 cups of assorted fresh mixed greens (such as, arugula, radicchio, baby spinach, watercress and romaine)
1 small red onion, thinly sliced and rings separated
20 firm cherry tomatoes, halved
1/4 cup chopped walnuts
1/4 cup dried cranberries
2 tablespoons of balsamic vinegar
4 teaspoons extra-virgin olive oil
1 tablespoon water
1/2 teaspoon of dried oregano, crushed
2 cloves garlic, finely minced
Crumbled feta cheese
Coarsely ground fresh pepper to taste

In a large salad bowl, combine greens, onion, tomatoes, walnuts, and cranberries. Gently toss. Dressing; combine vinegar, oil, water, oregano and garlic, shake well. Pour dressing over salad and toss lightly to coat. Garnish with feta cheese if desired and fresh pepper.

Approx. 140 calories
2g protein, 12g fat, 6g carbohydrates,
0mg cholesterol, 47mg sodium, 1g fiber

NORTH AFRICAN ZUCCHINI SALAD

Ingredients: Makes 4 servings

1 lb. of firm green zucchini, thinly sliced
Juice from 1 large lemon
2 cloves garlic, finely minced
1/2 teaspoon ground cumin
1 tablespoon of extra-virgin olive oil
1 1/2 tablespoons of plain low-fat yogurt
Salt and freshly ground black pepper to taste
Finely chopped parsley
Crumbled feta cheese

Steam zucchini until crispy tender (roughly 2-5 minutes). Rinse under cold water and drain well. In a large salad bowl mix the lemon juice, garlic, cumin, oil, yogurt and salt and pepper to taste. Add zucchini and gently toss. Chill in the refrigerator for 45 minutes to 1 hour before serving. Garnish with parsley and cheese if desired.

> *Approx. 66 calories per serving*
> *4g protein, 4g fat, 6g carbohydrates,*
> *0 cholesterol, 229 mg. sodium, 1g fiber*

GREENS WITH CHEESE MEDALLIONS

Ingredients: Makes 6 servings

6 cups (roughly 16-18 oz.) of mixed greens, such as escarole, red and green leaf lettuce, radicchio, and endive, washed and well dried.
6 oz. of soft goats cheese, log style
1/2 cup of extra-virgin olive oil
1/4 cup of plain bread crumbs
2 tablespoons freshly crushed garlic
Olive oil spray
1 cup halved cherry tomatoes
2 tablespoons of red wine vinegar
2 teaspoons of Dijon-style mustard
Salt and freshly ground black pepper to taste
Finely chopped pecans (optional)

Preheat broiler. Cut goat cheese log into 6 equal pieces and place cheese medallions in a bowl containing 1/4 cup olive oil, lightly swish mixture. Transfer the oil-laden cheese medallions to a bowl containing a mixture of breadcrumbs and crushed garlic. Coat medallions on both sides with breadcrumbs and garlic mixture. Lightly spray a baking sheet with olive oil spray and place medallions on sheet, broil until golden brown and crisp, 1-2 minutes per side. Toss greens with tomatoes, divide into 6 portions and top each portion with a cheese medallion. Combine the remaining oil, red wine vinegar, and Dijon mustard in a bottle and shake to mix well. Drizzle mixture over salads. Add salt and pepper to taste. Garnish with pecans if desired before serving.

Approx. 204 calories per serving
6g protein, 17g fat, 6g carbohydrates,
0 cholesterol, 159mg sodium, 1g fiber

FENNEL SALAD

Ingredients: Makes 4-6 servings

1 large clove garlic, halved
1 large fennel bulb, thinly sliced
1/2 English cucumber, thinly sliced
1 tablespoon minced fresh chives
8 large radishes, thinly slice
3 tablespoons of extra-virgin olive oil
2 1/2 tablespoons freshly squeezed lemon juice
Salt and freshly ground black pepper to taste
Marinated mixed olives (optional)

Rub the inside of a large bowl with garlic. Add fennel, cucumber, chives
and radishes. Whisk together olive oil, fresh lemon juice and salt and
pepper to taste. Pour olive oil mixture over salad and toss to mix.
Garnish with marinated olives if desired.

> *Approx. 76 calories per serving*
> *0 protein, 7g fat, 3g carbohydrates,*
> *2mg cholesterol, 20 mg sodium, 1g fiber*

TUNISIAN CARROT SALAD

Ingredients: Makes 6 servings

10 medium carrots, peeled and sliced into 1/2 inch-thick slices
5 teaspoons of freshly minced garlic
Salt to taste
2 teaspoons caraway seed
1 tablespoon of Harissa (recipe next page)
6 tablespoons of cider vinegar
1/4 cup extra-virgin olive oil
1 cup crumbled feta cheese
20 pitted Kalamata olives

In a medium saucepan filled with water cook carrots until tender. Drain and cool under cold running water, drain again and place in bowl.
Combine garlic, salt and caraway seed in a mortar and grind until it forms a rough paste. Pulse the ingredients in a food processor. Add Harissa and vinegar and mix well. Mash the carrots. Add the garlic-caraway mixture to Harissa blend well, mix in olive oil. Add 3/4 of the cheese and olives and toss again. Place salad in a shallow bowl and garnish with remaining feta cheese and olives.

Approx. 138 calories per serving
7g proteins, 7g fat, 13 carbohydrates,
0 cholesterol, 643mg sodium, 17g fiber

HARISSA PASTE (RED PEPPER SPICE)

Harissa paste is imported from North Africa in jars and tubes and is available in most specialty markets. To make Harissa yourself you will need.

1 oz. of hot red chili peppers
1 teaspoon caraway seed
1/2 teaspoon cumin seed
1/2 teaspoon coriander seed
2 garlic cloves, peeled
1/4 teaspoon salt
1 tablespoon water
4 tablespoons extra-virgin olive oil

Soak red peppers in a bowl of hot water for 1 hour. Meanwhile grind the spices together in a spice mill. Drain peppers, pat dry and chop. Place in a mortar with garlic, spices, and salt and mix into a paste. Add water and olive oil, mix well and store paste in a jar. Refrigerate. Paste keeps for months.

> *Approx. 37 calories per 1 teaspoon serving*
> *0 protein, 4g fat, 1g carbohydrate, 0 cholesterol, 34mg sodium, 0 fiber*

CLASSIC GREEK SALAD

Ingredients: Makes 6 servings

1/4 cup of extra-virgin olive oil
3 tablespoons red wine vinegar
2 cloves garlic, finely minced
Pinch of sugar or Splenda
1 tablespoon dried oregano
Salt and fresh black pepper to taste
1/2 head of escarole, shredded
6 large firm tomatoes, quartered
1/2 English cucumber, peeled, seeded, thinly sliced into
1 medium red bell pepper, seeded, sliced
1/2 red onion, sliced
1/2 lb. Greek feta cheese, cut into small cube
20 Greek black olives
1/4 cup freshly chopped Italian parsley

Whisk together oil, vinegar, garlic, oregano, sugar, salt and black pepper. Set aside. Combine escarole, tomatoes, cucumbers, pepper, onion, and cheese in a large salad bowl and toss together. Drizzle oil mixture over salad and toss. Scatter olives and parsley over salad and serve.

> **Approx. 268 calories per serving**
> **23g protein, 38g fat, 44g carbohydrates,**
> **0 cholesterol, 595mg sodium, 3g fiber**

LIGHT CAESAR SALAD

Ingredients: Makes 6 servings

1-2 bunches packaged pre-cleaned romaine lettuce, torn in pieces
1/2 cup of non-fat plain yogurt
2 teaspoons lemon juice
2 1/2 teaspoons of balsamic vinegar
1 teaspoon Worcestershire sauce
2 cloves freshly minced garlic
1/2 teaspoon anchovy paste
1/2 cup grated Parmesan cheese
10 small pitted black olives, chopped

Clean and pat dry romaine lettuce and place in large salad bowl. In blender mix yogurt, lemon juice, vinegar, Worcestershire sauce, garlic, anchovy paste and 1/4 cup Parmesan cheese until smooth. Pour mixture over lettuce and toss. Garnish with remaining cheese and olives

> *Approx. 49 calories per serving*
> *4g protein, 1g fat, 4g carbohydrates,*
> *4 mg cholesterol, 112 mg. Sodium, 1g fiber*

MOROCCAN EGGPLANT SALAD

Ingredients: Makes 4 servings

1 large unpeeled eggplant (about 1 lb.) cubed
3 cloves garlic, finely chopped
5 cups water
1 teaspoon salt
3 tablespoons extra-virgin olive oil
2 large tomatoes, chopped
1 teaspoon cumin
1 teaspoon paprika
1/4 cup lemon juice

In a pot, place the eggplant cubes, roughly 1/3 of garlic, water, and salt. Cover and boil for about 5-10 minutes or until the eggplant is cooked but still firm. Drain cubes in a strainer and allow too cool. In a large skillet, heat 2 tablespoons olive oil. Add tomatoes, remaining garlic, cumin and paprika. Stir while mashing with a fork until mixture is somewhat smooth. Remove from heat. Combine eggplant cubes with tomato mixture in a bowl, allow to slightly cool before covering. Refrigerate and chill for about 2 hours before serving. Before serving, add lemon juice and remainder of olive oil and gently toss.

Approx: 128 calories per serving
1g protein, 7g fat, 13g carbohydrates,
0 cholesterol, 561mg sodium, 4g fiber

SYRIAN CUCUMBER AND YOGURT SALAD

Ingredients: Makes 4 servings

1 1/2 teaspoons freshly crushed garlic
1/8 teaspoon minced fresh dill
Salt to taste
1 quart plain low-fat yogurt
2 English cucumbers, peeled and diced
2 tablespoons dried mint

In a bowl combine garlic, dill and salt. Add yogurt and mix well. Stir in cucumbers and mint. Cover and refrigerator until well chilled before serving.

> *Approx: 167 calories per serving*
> *13g protein, 4g fat, 21g carbohydrates,*
> *10 mg cholesterol, 183 mg sodium, 1g fiber*

TUNISIAN TUNA SALAD

Ingredients: Makes 4 servings

3 large ripe tomatoes, peeled
2 medium green bell peppers, seeded and sliced into thin rings
1 large cucumber, sliced
1 sweet onion, thinly sliced and separated into rings
2 hard-boiled eggs, shelled and divided into quarters
2 tablespoons fresh lemon juice
2 cloves garlic, minced
2 tablespoons of red wine vinegar
1 tablespoon water
1 teaspoon Dijon mustard
2 tablespoons chopped fresh basil
1/4 cup extra-virgin olive oil
1(12 oz.) can of water packed white albacore, drained and divided into 4 equal parts
Salt and freshly cracked black pepper to taste
1 tablespoon capers, rinsed and well drained
Chopped Kalamata olives

Divide tomatoes, peppers, cucumbers, onion rings and eggs into 4 portions. On 4 individual salad platters first layer tomatoes then cover with layers of pepper rings, cucumbers, and onions. Arrange eggs around edges of platters. In a small bowl, whisk the lemon juice, garlic, vinegar, water, mustard and basil together until smooth. Gradually whisk in olive oil. Pour dressing over each salad platter. Place a scoop of tuna on the center of each salad. Add salt and cracked pepper to taste. Garnish with capers and olives.

Approx: 306 calories per serving
27g protein, 17g fat, 13g carbohydrates,
132mg cholesterol, 332mg sodium, 3g fiber

FRESHLY CHOPPED SALAD WITH WALNUT DRESSING

Ingredients: Makes 6 servings

3 medium ripe tomatoes, seeded and chopped
1 medium cucumber, peeled, seeded and diced
1 large green bell pepper, seeded and diced
5 scallions, finely chopped
1 head Butter head lettuce, clean and separate leaves
20 pitted Kalamata black olives
1/4 cup finely chopped fresh spearmint leaves

For Walnut Dressing-
1/4 cup shelled walnuts, finely minced
2 slices of Italian bread, soaked in water, squeezed dry, and crumbled
1/2 teaspoon of finely crushed garlic
1/4 cup extra-virgin olive oil
Lemon juice, freshly squeezed, to taste
Salt to taste
Red hot pepper sauce to taste

In a large mixing bowl combine tomatoes, cucumber, and green pepper and chopped scallions. Add Walnut dressing and toss thoroughly. Add salt to taste. Line a serving platter with lettuce leaves. With a large spoon, spoon salad mixture over lettuce leaves, sprinkle with mint and garnish with olives. Serve immediately.

Walnut Dressing- In a blender or food processor add bread, walnuts and garlic and blend while slowly adding olive oil. Gradually add lemon juice and beat until mixture is smooth. Add salt and hot pepper sauce to taste.

> *Approx. 195 calories per serving of salad plus dressing*
> *4g protein, 16g fat, 13g carbohydrates,*
> *0 cholesterol, 227mg sodium, 3g fiber*

SIMPLE SPANISH SALAD

Ingredients: Makes 6 servings

1 bag (2 bunches) cleaned and trimmed romaine lettuce, torn into bite sized pieces
3 medium ripe tomatoes cut into 1/4-inch wedges
1 large sweet onion, thinly sliced
1 green pepper, seeded, thinly sliced
1 red pepper, seeded, thinly sliced
1/4 cup chopped marinated green olives
1/4 cup chopped black olives
1/4 cup extra-virgin olive oil
3 tablespoons balsamic vinegar

Use six chilled salad plates, placing a bed of romaine on each plate. Arrange tomatoes, onions, peppers, and olives on the top of the lettuce on each plate. Mix olive oil and vinegar together, drizzle over salad. Serve salad chilled.

> *Approx. 107 calories per serving*
> *2g protein, 9g fat, 7g carbohydrates,*
> *0 cholesterol, 145mg sodium, 3g fiber*

EASY COUSCOUS PARSLEY SALAD

Ingredients: Makes 4 servings

1/4 cup couscous
1/4 cup water
2 tablespoons fresh lemon juice
2 teaspoons extra-virgin olive oil
1/4 cup fresh flat parsley leaves, finely chopped
2 tablespoons finely chopped fresh mint leaves
2 teaspoons lemon rinds, finely chopped
2 tablespoons pine nuts
Salt and freshly ground black pepper to taste
1 medium ripe tomato, peeled, seeded
2 heads Belgian endive, leaves for scooping
Whole wheat pita rounds, cut into wedges and toasted until crispy
(optional)

Combine couscous with water and lemon in a medium bowl and let stand for 1 hour. After 1 hour, add olive oil, parsley, mint, lemon rind, pine nuts, salt, and pepper to taste. Mix well. Mold couscous mixture into a mound in the center of a serving platter and garnish with tomato. Surround with endive leaves or toasted pita wedges if desired. Serve at room temperature.

Approx. 120 calories per serving
5g protein, 2g fat, 18g carbohydrate,
0 cholesterol, 65mg sodium, 9g fiber

SARDINE SALAD

Ingredients: Makes 4-6 servings

8 oz. of a spiral shaped pasta
1/4 cup extra-virgin olive oil
1 medium onion, thinly sliced
2 cloves fresh garlic, minced
1/2 of a small hot pepper, seeded and finely chopped
1/3 cup fresh squeezed orange juice
1/4 cup golden raisins
1/4 cup toasted sliced almonds
16 jumbo pitted green olives, chopped
9 oz. (2 cans) sardines in olive oil
Salt and freshly ground black pepper to taste
Splash of lemon juice
4 tablespoons finely chopped fresh parsley
Finely shredded Parmesan cheese

Cook pasta until tender, drain and set aside. Heat olive oil in a large skillet; add onions, garlic and hot peppers, sauté until golden brown. Add orange juice and raisins, bring to a boil. Remove from heat but keep warm. Combine toasted almonds and olives with onion mixture, stir together. Add sardines but try not to break into pieces. Pour sardine mixture over pasta. Add salt and pepper to taste, and a splash of lemon juice. Garnish with parsley and a small amount of cheese. Serve at room temperature.

> **Approx. 467 calories per serving**
> **31g protein, 26g fat, 38g carbohydrates,**
> **60mg cholesterol, 288 mg sodium, 1g fiber**

AVOCADO SALAD

Ingredients: Makes 3 (1 cup) servings

1 large ripe avocado, pitted and peeled
1 cup halved cherry tomatoes
1 small onion, finely chopped
2 tablespoons chopped fresh parsley
1/2 small hot pepper, finely chopped (optional)
2 teaspoons fresh lime juice
Salt and freshly ground black pepper to taste

Cut avocado into bite sized chunks. Combine tomatoes, parsley, onion, hot pepper and lime juice. Toss well, add salt and pepper to taste. Add avocado and gently toss. Divide into 3 equal servings and serve.

> *Approx: 130 calories per serving*
> *2g protein, 10g fat, 10g carbohydrates,*
> *0 cholesterol, 110mg sodium, 4g fiber*

SOUP

BASIC LENTIL SOUP

Ingredients: 6-8 servings

4 cups low-sodium chicken broth
4 cups water
1 cup split brown lentils, rinsed and drained
Salt and freshly ground black pepper to taste
2 teaspoons ground cumin
1/4 cup extra-virgin olive oil
2 medium yellow onions, finely chopped
4 large cloves garlic, finely chopped
2 oz. dry Ditalini pasta
1 large firm ripe tomato, seeded cut into chunks
10 oz. fresh escarole, washed and chopped
1 cup finely chopped parsley
1/2 cup fresh lemon juice
Shredded Parmesan cheese

In a large pot add chicken broth and water, bring to a boil. Add lentils, salt and pepper and cumin, reduce heat to medium and cook until lentils are tender. Do not over cook, beans should be tender but firm. While lentils are cooking, add oil to a skillet and sauté onions and garlic until golden brown. Stir mixture often to prevent burning, when browned, set aside. When lentils are almost tender add pasta and cook until both are tender but not mushy, reduce heat to low-simmer add garlic mixture, tomatoes, chopped escarole, parsley and lemon juice. Simmer until escarole is cooked. Serve garnished with a small amount of cheese.

Approx. 195 calories per serving
8g protein, 11g fat, 26g carbohydrates,
3mg cholesterol, 152mg sodium, 6g fiber

SAVORY MEDITERRANEAN CHICKPEA SOUP

Ingredients: 6 servings

2 cups of water
4 cups low-sodium chicken broth
4 cups canned chickpeas, rinsed with fresh water and drained
1 tablespoon extra-virgin olive oil
1 large onion, chopped
4-5 cloves fresh garlic minced
1 medium green pepper, chopped
1 teaspoon cayenne
2 teaspoons dried sage
2 teaspoons dried rosemary
1 teaspoon ground cinnamon
Salt and freshly ground black pepper to taste
1/4 cup crumbled low-fat crumbled feta cheese (optional)
2 tablespoons fresh parsley, finely chopped

In a large pot combine water, broth, chickpeas, olive oil, onion, garlic, green pepper, cayenne, sage, rosemary, and cinnamon. Bring mixture to boil over medium heat, lower temperature and simmer for 20 minutes, uncovered. Add salt and pepper to taste. Garnish with feta cheese and parsley.

> *Approx. 163 calories per serving*
> *9g protein, 3g fat, 32g carbohydrates,*
> *3mg cholesterol, 560mg sodium, 8g fiber*

FRESH GARDEN GAZPACHO

Ingredients: 4 servings

4 cups chopped ripe tomatoes, peeled
4 cloves garlic, chopped
1/2 red onion, chopped
1 green pepper, seeded, diced
1/4 cup extra-virgin olive oil
2 tablespoons red wine vinegar
2 slices stale French sourdough bread
1/2 cup canned tomato juice
1/2 teaspoon cumin
1/2 small hot pepper, finely chopped
1 tablespoon chopped fresh basil
Salt and freshly ground black pepper to taste
Finely diced green peppers and cucumbers
Croutons (optional)
Low-fat sour cream or yogurt (optional)

In a food processor or blender, add tomatoes, garlic, onion and green pepper. Blend until pureed. Add olive oil and vinegar, blend about 1 minute to mix. Soak bread in tomato juice, add soaked bread mixture to blender. Add cumin, hot peppers and basil. Blend for 2-3 minutes to mix well. Adjust with salt and pepper to taste. Chill for several hours. Serve very chilled, garnished with diced green peppers and cucumber. If desired, add croutons and a dollop of sour cream or yogurt.

> *Approx. 210 calories per serving*
> *4g protein, 15g fat, 20g carbohydrates,*
> *0 cholesterol, 201 mg sodium, 3g fiber*

ITALIAN MINESTRONE SOUP WITH PESTO

Ingredients: 6-8 servings

1 cup dried cannellini beans
4 cups low-sodium chicken broth
4 cups water
2 medium white potatoes, peeled and diced
2 oz. dry Ditalini pasta
2 large carrots, chopped
3 stalks celery, chopped
1/2 cup chopped white onion
2 cloves garlic, minced
1 cup tomato juice
3 plum tomatoes, chopped
1 large zucchini, chopped
Freshly shredded Parmesan cheese

For pesto:
1 cup fresh basil leaves
1 teaspoon dried basil leaves, crumbled
4 cloves garlic, finely minced
3 tablespoons extra-virgin olive oil
1/2 cup grated Parmesan cheese
Salt and freshly ground black pepper to taste

Rinse dried Cannellini beans and place in a large covered pot. Add chicken broth and water and bring to a boil. Uncover pot, reduce heat and simmer until beans are tender. Roughly 1 hour. Add potatoes, pasta, carrots, celery, onion, and garlic and tomato juice. Return mixture to a boil, then reduce heat and simmer uncovered for 10 minutes.

(Continued)

Add tomatoes and zucchini, simmer until all are tender. Process pesto ingredients in a food processor or blender until finely chopped. Remove soup from heat and stir in pesto mixture and serve garnished with Parmesan cheese

Approx. 182 calories per serving without pesto
10g protein, 1g fat, 20g carbohydrates,
3 mg cholesterol, 204mg sodium, 4g fiber

Approx. 254 calories per serving with pesto added
12g protein, 8g fat, 20g carbohydrates,
10mg cholesterol, 291mg sodium, 4g fiber

FRENCH PISTOU SOUP

Ingredients: 6 servings

1 tablespoon extra-virgin olive oil
1 medium onion, finely chopped
1/2 cup dry kidney beans
2 medium potatoes, diced
1 stalk celery, chopped
2 cups chopped carrots
8 cups of water
8 oz. fresh green beans cut in 1 inch pieces
1 leek, green part only, thinly sliced
2 medium tomatoes, peeled and chopped
2 small zucchini cut in 1 inch cubes
1 cup uncooked whole wheat elbow macaroni
Salt and freshly ground black pepper to taste

For pistou mix:
3 cloves garlic
2 cups fresh basil leaves
1 tablespoon of hot liquid from soup
Salt and freshly ground black pepper to taste
3 tablespoons extra-virgin olive oil
Freshly grated Gruyere cheese for garnish

In large saucepan heat oil, add onion, cook to soften. Add kidney beans, potatoes, celery, carrots and 8 cups of water. Bring to a boil, reduce heat, simmer covered, for about 15 minutes. Add green beans, leek, tomatoes, zucchini and pasta, cook another 10 minutes or until the vegetables are tender. Season mixture with salt and pepper to taste. Reduce heat to very-low, cover to keep warm.

(Continued)

Make Pistou: In a food processor, finely chopped garlic and basil. Add soup liquid, salt and pepper to taste and oil. Ladle soup into individual soup bowls, spoon in some pistou and garnish with cheese.

Approx. 248 calories per serving
10g protein, 9g fat, 35 g carbohydrates,
0 cholesterol, 28mg sodium, 8g fiber

EGG-LEMON PASTA SOUP

Ingredients: 4 servings

4 cups low-sodium chicken broth
4 oz. Ditalini pasta
1/2 cup egg substitute or 2 large whole eggs if desired
1/2 cup fresh lemon juice
Salt and freshly ground black pepper to taste
4 tablespoons chopped fresh parsley
1 lemon, thinly sliced

In a medium saucepan, bring chicken broth to a boil. Add pasta; return to a boil stirring once. Reduce to low; simmer 3-5 minutes. Remove from heat. Beat the eggs in a bowl and beat in the lemon juice. Add a ladle of soup to this mixture and stir then transfer to soup pot. Heat soup on low-heat, do not curdle the eggs. Add salt and pepper to taste. Divide soup into 4 portions, garnish with parsley and lemon slices and serve.

> *Approx. 161 calories per serving*
> *10g protein, 2g fat, 65g carbohydrates,*
> *5mg cholesterol, 197mg sodium, 1g fiber*

CHILLY TOMATO SOUP

Ingredients- 4 servings

10 medium ripe tomatoes
1/2 tablespoon extra-virgin olive oil
4-5 cloves garlic, minced
2 tablespoons chopped onions
2 cups low-sodium chicken broth
2 teaspoons Splenda (when cooking with Splenda, use boxed Splenda Granular)
1/2 teaspoon fresh basil
Salt and freshly ground black pepper to taste

For garnish:
8 scallions, chopped (optional)
2 cucumbers, diced (optional)
1 large green zucchini, diced (optional)

In a large pot of boiling water dip tomatoes for 30 seconds then immediately place tomatoes in cold water. Allow to sit until they can be handled. Skin tomatoes with a paring knife, cut tomatoes in half crosswise and remove seeds. Core and then cut into quarter pieces. In a blender or food processor process tomatoes until pureed. In a skillet; heat olive oil and sauté garlic and onions until tender. Remove from heat. In a large bowl combine pureed tomatoes, sautéed onion mixture, chicken broth, Splenda, basil, salt and pepper, stirring to incorporate.   Refrigerate soup for 4-6 hours until well chilled. Garnish with scallions, cucumbers and zucchini if desired.

> **Approx. 69 calories per serving**
> **6g protein, 3g fat, 13g carbohydrates,**
> **1mg cholesterol, 106 mg sodium, 4g fiber**

CHUNKY CHICKEN AND CABBAGE SOUP

Ingredients: 4-6 servings

4 cups low-sodium chicken broth
2 cups water
8 oz. skinless, boneless chicken, cubed
2 medium potatoes, peeled and chunked
1 cup chopped carrots
2 bay leaves
4-6 whole peppercorns
1/2 teaspoon cumin
1 cup chopped celery
1 medium onion, chunked
3 cloves garlic, chopped
1 small head of cabbage, torn
2 medium tomatoes, peeled and quartered
1/4 cup parsley, finely chopped
Salt and pepper to taste
Garnish with 1 tablespoon of non-fat yogurt (optional)

In a large pot, bring chicken broth, water, chicken, potatoes, carrots, bay leaves, peppercorns and cumin to boil. Reduce heat, simmer for 30-40 minutes or until chicken is cooked. Add celery, onion, garlic, cabbage, tomatoes and parsley, cook for additional 15 minutes or until vegetables are tender. Add salt and pepper to taste. Garnish each serving with yogurt if desired.

> Approx. 143 calories per serving
> 15g protein, 2g fat, 21g carbohydrates,
> 21mg cholesterol, 50mg sodium, 3g fiber

HEARTY BEAN SOUP

Ingredients: 6-8 servings

2 cups water
2 medium potatoes, peeled, coarsely chopped
2 large carrots, coarsely chopped
2 stalks celery, coarsely chopped
1 bay leaf
1 tablespoon fresh thyme
Salt and freshly ground black pepper to taste
3 tablespoons extra-virgin olive oil
5 cloves fresh garlic, minced
1 medium onion, finely chopped
1/2 small hot pepper, finely chopped
5 cups low-sodium chicken broth
4 (15 oz.) cans Great Northern Beans
Salt and freshly ground black pepper to taste
Grated Parmesan cheese (optional)
Chopped fresh flat leaf parsley (optional)

In a heavy pot, combine water, potato, carrots, celery, bay leaf, thyme, salt and pepper. Bring to a boil, reduce heat, cover and simmer until vegetables are tender. While vegetables are cooking, combine in a large skillet, oil, garlic, onion and hot peppers, sauté until tender and lightly browned. Add to garlic mixture, 1 cup of chicken broth and beans, mix together well, cover and simmer for about 10 minutes to allow for flavors to blend. Add salt and pepper to taste. Combine bean mixture and 4 cups of chicken broth and to vegetable pot. Stir to mix, keep at a low simmer for about 10-15 minutes, allowing flavors to blend. Garnish with cheese and parsley, if desired.

Approx. 220 calories
11g protein, 6g fat, 36g carbohydrates,
3mg cholesterol, 663 mg sodium, 9g fiber

SPINACH FETA CHEESE SOUP

Ingredients: 6-8 servings

10 oz. spinach, washed under running water
6 cups low-sodium chicken broth
1/4 cup fresh cilantro, chopped
2 tablespoons extra-virgin olive oil
1 large white onion, coarsely chopped
2 medium potatoes, peeled and diced
4 cloves fresh garlic, minced
1 teaspoon ground cumin
1 (10 oz.) package frozen baby lima beans, thawed
1/3 cup couscous
6 oz. feta cheese, cut into chunks
1/2 teaspoon freshly ground black pepper to taste
Finely chopped parsley
Lemon wedges

Cut half of the spinach leaves into thin ribbons, reserving stems. Set aside. Using a food processor or blender, combine the reserved stems and the remaining spinach with 1 cup of broth, and the cilantro. Process until smooth and set aside. In a large pot, heat olive oil over medium heat, add onion, sauté until golden brown then add potatoes, garlic and cumin, stir to make sure potatoes are well coated. Add remaining 5 cups of broth. Reduce heat to medium and cook until potatoes are tender, roughly 15 minutes. Add ribbon spinach, spinach-cilantro puree, lima beans, couscous and cheese. Cook until lima beans are crispy tender and cheese has melted through soup. Season soup, with fresh ground pepper. Divide soup into 6 servings. For garnish, sprinkle parsley over soup and add a lemon wedge on the side.

Approx. 226 calories per serving
10g protein, 10g fat, 24g carbohydrates,
15mg cholesterol, 157mg sodium, 4g fiber

CHUNKY FISH CHOWDER WITH SAFFRON

Ingredients: Makes 6 servings

1 pound fresh Grouper fillets
1 pound fresh tuna or Cod fillets
2 tablespoons extra-virgin olive oil
8-10 diced scallions
1 cup chopped celery
3 large cloves garlic, crushed
1 small yellow pepper, diced
1 small red pepper, diced
1 teaspoon turmeric
1/4 teaspoon ground saffron
1 1/4 cup dry white wine
8 oz. bottled clam juice
4 cups water
2 bay leaves
1/2 teaspoon thyme
1/4 teaspoon crushed red hot pepper flakes
Salt to taste
3/4 cup small elbow macaroni, uncooked
2 tablespoons lemon juice
4 tablespoons chopped fresh parsley

(Continued)

Rinse and cut fish fillets into 1-inch cubes, refrigerate. In a large heavy bottom skillet; heat olive oil and sauté onions, celery, garlic and peppers. Add turmeric and saffron and cook additional few more minutes. Stir in wine, clam juice and water. Add in bay leaves, thyme, red pepper flakes and salt. Bring to boil and reduce heat to simmer for 10 minutes. Add pasta and cook until pasta is tender. Add fish and simmer for 10-15 minutes longer until fish is cooked. Remove bay leaves. Add lemon juice, stir to mix. Serve garnished with parsley.

Approx. 296 calories per serving
35g protein, 8g fat, 11g carbohydrates, 27mg cholesterol,
187 mg sodium, 3g fiber

CHICKEN ESCAROLE SOUP

Ingredients: Makes 4-6 servings

3 cups water (enough to cover chicken)
5 skinless, boneless chicken breasts; cut into chunks
1 small white onion cut in half
1/8 cup black peppercorns
1 bay leaf
4 cloves fresh garlic, finely minced
3 cups low-salt chicken broth
2 medium sized carrots, sliced
1 celery stalk, sliced
1/2 head escarole, cut into 1-inch strips, stems removed
Salt and freshly ground black pepper to taste
Freshly grated Parmesan cheese for garnish

In a large saucepan, combine water, chicken, onion, peppercorns, bay leaf, and garlic. Bring to a boil, reduce heat to low, cover and simmer 1 hour or until chicken is tender. Remove chicken from broth and strain out bay leaf and peppercorns, set aside. In a separate saucepan, combine canned chicken broth with strained broth, add carrots and celery, bring to a rapid boil, reduce to low and simmer for 10 minutes or until vegetables are crispy tender. Stir in escarole and chicken, heat through add salt and pepper to taste and serve. Garnish each serving with a sprinkling of grated cheese.

> **Approx: 153 calories per serving**
> **28g protein, 2g fat, 4g carbohydrates,**
> **62mg cholesterol, 129mg sodium, 5g fiber**

CHILLED CUCUMBER SOUP

Ingredients: Makes 4-6 servings

2 large English cucumbers, peeled and coarsely chopped
1 medium yellow onion, coarsely chopped
5 cups low-sodium chicken broth
2 cups plain low-fat yogurt
2 scallions, finely minced (white and green parts)
Salt and freshly ground black pepper to taste
Fresh dill, finely chopped

Combine cucumber and onion in a large saucepan, add chicken broth. Heat on high heat to rapid boil, immediately reduce to simmer, cover and simmer until vegetables are just tender. Remove from heat, allow too cool slightly then refrigerate to chill for several hours. To serve, blend in yogurt, scallions and salt to taste. Sprinkle with fresh cracked pepper and dill.

Approx: 91 calories per serving
7g protein, 3g fat, 10g carbohydrates, 4mg cholesterol,
164 mg sodium, 1g fiber

EGGPLANT SOUP

Ingredients: Makes 4-6 servings

2 tablespoons extra-virgin olive oil
2 cloves fresh garlic, minced
1/2 medium onion thinly sliced, rings separated
1 medium eggplant, peeled and cut into 1/2 inch cubes
1/2 teaspoon oregano
1/4 teaspoon thyme
4 cups low-sodium chicken broth
1/2 cup dry sherry
Salt and freshly ground black pepper to taste
1 large tomato, sliced
10 oz. non-fat feta cheese, crumbled
Freshly grated Parmesan cheese (optional)

Heat oil in large skillet over medium heat; add garlic and onion, sauté until lightly golden. Add eggplant, oregano and thyme; continue cooking until eggplant browns slightly, stirring constantly. Reduce heat to low, add broth, cover and simmer for roughly 5 minutes. Add sherry, cover, and continue to simmer for another 2-3 minutes. Stir in salt and pepper to taste if needed and remove from heat. Allow too cool slightly. Pre-heat broiler, pour slightly cooled soup into an oven-proof bowl. Top soup with tomato slices and feta cheese, place soup under broiler and heat until feta melts into soup. Garnish with grated Parmesan cheese, if desired and broil until cheese is browned.

> **Approx; 146 calories per serving**
> **9g protein, 6g fat, 10g carbohydrates, 3mg cholesterol,**
> **538mg sodium, 2g fiber**

PIZZA

In the Mediterranean regions, a pizza made at home is a well-balanced modern meal, as opposed to the fast food pizza served in the United States. A Mediterranean home style pizza is made from complex carbohydrate pizza dough, fresh vegetables, small amounts of animal protein, and monounsaturated fat in the form of extra-virgin olive oil. In contrast, the pizza made in the United States is loaded with saturated fat, sugar and sodium.

TOMATO EGGPLANT AND BASIL PIZZA

Ingredients: Makes enough for 15-inch crust (8 slices)

Crispy thin whole wheat pizza crust (page 120)
1 large eggplant
6 garlic cloves, minced
2 tablespoons extra-virgin olive oil
5 medium tomatoes, seeded and chopped
3 tablespoons fresh basil, chopped
Pinch hot pepper flakes
3 cups crumbled non-fat feta cheese
Salt and ground black pepper to taste
1/3 cup freshly grated Parmesan cheese and fresh rosemary, finely chopped (optional)

Preheat oven to 425 degrees F. Follow directions for pizza dough and roll out to a 12-15-inch round. Place pizza round on scantly oiled pizza pan. Cut eggplant in half the long way, slash down the middle but not through skin. Place on pan and bake for 20- 30 minutes. Skin should be shriveled and eggplant tender. Remove to a plate and reserve, when cooled, slice crosswise into thin slices. Sauté garlic in 1 tablespoon of olive oil over low heat, until softened. Add tomatoes, basil, and hot pepper flakes. Brush pizza dough lightly with 1/2 teaspoon olive oil, top with tomato mixture then feta cheese and arrange eggplant slices in pinwheel pattern, slightly overlapping the slices. Season pizza with salt and pepper and drizzle remaining olive oil over eggplant. Bake at 425 degrees F. for 10 to 15 minutes until pizza crust is brown and crisp. Garnish top of pizza with Parmesan cheese and rosemary if desired.

Approx. 166 calories per slice
20g protein, 2g fat, 21g carbohydrates,
0 cholesterol, 1385mg sodium, 1g fiber

PIZZA MARGHERITA

Ingredients: Makes enough for 15-inch crust (8 slices)

Thin pizza dough (page 122)
4 Roma tomatoes, thinly sliced
Salt and freshly ground pepper to taste
1/2 cup thinly sliced yellow sweet pepper
3/4 cup shredded part-skim mozzarella cheese, about 3 oz.
4-5 snipped fresh basil leaves
1/4 cup freshly grated Parmesan cheese
1 tablespoon extra-virgin olive oil

Preheat oven to 450 degrees. Follow directions for pizza dough and roll out to a 12-15-inch round. Place dough on a scantly oiled pizza pan. Spread tomatoes on rolled out dough almost to the edge of the crust. Sprinkle with salt and pepper to taste. Top tomatoes with yellow peppers, mozzarella cheese, basil, Parmesan cheese and drizzle olive oil over the top. Bake at 450 degrees for 8-10 minutes or until crust is golden brown and cheeses are melted.

> *Approx. 202 calories per slice*
> *11g protein, 7g fat, 28g carbohydrates,*
> *7mg cholesterol, 375mg sodium, 1g fiber*

SPICY SWEET PEPPER PIZZA

Ingredients: Makes enough for 15-inch crust (8 slices)

Whole wheat pizza dough (page 121)
1 tablespoon extra-virgin olive oil
3 large red peppers, seeded and thinly sliced
3 large yellow peppers, seeded and thinly sliced
2 cloves garlic, minced
1 tablespoon fresh thyme, chopped
Salt and freshly ground pepper to taste
Hot pepper flakes to taste
1 cup shredded part-skim mozzarella cheese

Preheat oven for 500 degrees. Follow directions for pizza dough and roll out to 12-15-inch round. Place dough on scantly oiled pizza pan. Heat oil in heavy bottomed pan and sauté the peppers and garlic, about 10 minutes until soft. Stir in thyme, salt and pepper to taste and red pepper flakes. Preheat oven to 500 degrees. Spread pepper mixture over pizza dough, sprinkle cheese over pepper mixture bake for 20 to 25 minutes until crust is golden browned and cheese has melted.

> *Approx. 209 calories per slice*
> *9g protein, 7g fat, 25g carbohydrates,*
> *7mg cholesterol, 78mg sodium, 4g fiber*

WILD MUSHROOM PIZZA

Ingredients: Makes enough for 15-inch crust (8 slices)

Thin crust pizza dough (page 122)
3 oz. dried Porcine mushrooms
1 quart warm water
2 tablespoons extra-virgin olive oil
4 cloves garlic, finely minced
1 cup fresh button mushrooms, cleaned and thinly sliced
1 cup fresh shiitakes or other wild mushroom
4 tablespoons white wine
1 tablespoon soy sauce
1/2 teaspoon dries thyme
1/2 teaspoon dried rosemary
Salt and freshly ground pepper to taste
3 tablespoons chopped fresh parsley
8 oz. shredded smoked provolone cheese

Preheat oven to 425 degrees. Follow directions for pizza dough, when ready, roll it out to a 15-inch round. Place on scantly oiled pizza pan. Soak the dried mushrooms in warm water for 30 minutes. After soaking, squeeze mushrooms of excess liquid and chop coarsely. Strain soaking water through a cheesecloth and set aside. Heat 1 tablespoon of olive oil over medium heat in a heavy bottomed skillet and add half of the garlic. Sauté garlic, stirring often until it becomes golden. Add both dried and fresh mushrooms, sauté for about 5 minutes until they begin to release their liquid and add wine and soy sauce. Continue to sauté until wine evaporates. Add soaking liquid to mushrooms, thyme, rosemary, remaining garlic, salt and pepper to taste. Increase heat; continue cooking and stirring until most of the liquid has evaporated and mushrooms have

(Continued)

become glazed. Add parsley and remove from heat. Brush pizza dough with remaining olive oil. Evenly spread cheese over crust. Spread mushroom mixture over cheese and bake for roughly 8-10 minutes, until crust is golden brown and crisp and cheese is melted.

Approx. 208 calories per slice
9g protein, 10g fat, 22g carbohydrates,
0 cholesterol, 351mg sodium, 2g fiber

SUNDRIED TOMATO AND ANCHOVY PIZZA

Ingredients: Makes enough for 15-inch crust (8 slices)

Crispy thin whole wheat pizza crust (page 120)
1 red onion thinly sliced
8 sundried tomatoes in oil, chopped
1 tablespoon basil leaves, broken in pieces
1 can (2 oz.) anchovy fillets, chopped, sliced and oil reserved
1 clove garlic, minced
1 cup fresh part-skim mozzarella cheese, shredded
Salt and pepper to taste
Finely chopped fresh parsley for garnish (optional)

Preheat oven to 425 degrees. Follow directions for pizza dough, when ready, roll out to 15-inch round. Place on scantly oiled pizza pan. Top pizza crust dough, with onions, sundried tomatoes, basil, anchovies, garlic and fresh mozzarella. Salt and pepper to taste and bake at 425 degrees until crust is crisp and cheese is melted. Garnish with parsley if desired.

> *Approx: 137 calories per slice*
> *6g protein, 3g fat, 18g carbohydrates,*
> *10mg cholesterol, 119mg sodium, 1g fiber*

PROVENCAL VEGETABLE PIZZA

Ingredients: Makes 2 crusts (each 6 slices)

Pizza crust:
2 3/4 cups unbleached stone-ground white flour
2 teaspoons sea salt
1 envelope active dry yeast
1/2 teaspoon granulated sugar
3/4 cup lukewarm milk
2 large eggs, lightly beaten
1/2 stick, unsalted butter
2 tablespoons mixed chopped herbs (parsley, thyme, rosemary, basil and oregano)

Ratatouille filling:
2 tablespoons extra-virgin olive oil
1 small onion, chopped
3 cloves garlic, chopped
1 large red pepper, seeded and diced
5 medium tomatoes, peeled, seeded and diced
1 medium eggplant, cut into strips (1/4 x 2-inches)
2 medium zucchini, cut into strips (1/4 x 2-inches)
2 teaspoons chopped fresh thyme
Sea salt and fresh ground pepper to taste
2 oz. Gruyere cheese, shredded
2 large eggs
1/2 cup heavy cream

To make pizza crusts: In a medium-sized bowl, mix flour and salt. Make a well in the center of the flour. In a small bowl mix yeast, sugar and 1/4 cup milk, let stand until foamy. Add remaining milk. Whisk eggs into yeast mixture until well blended. Pour yeast mixture into the well of flour. Gradually work in flour from sides, beating until dough is smooth,

(Continued)

soft and slightly sticky. Knead the dough by pulling it up with fingers and down again into bowl with heel of hand until it is very smooth and elastic. Beat in the butter and herbs until there are no streaks of butter or herbs. Shape dough into a ball and place in a dry but oiled bowl. Cover and allow dough to rise at room temperature until it doubles, about 2 hours.

To make filling: In large skillet heat oil add onion and garlic, cook until tender, but not browned. Add red pepper, cook for about 5 minutes stirring frequently. Stir in tomatoes, eggplant, zucchini, thyme, and salt and pepper. Cook about 10 minutes or until vegetables are tender but not mushy. Let cool. Preheat oven to 400 degrees.

When dough is ready, turn out onto a floured board and divide into two equal portions. Roll out each ball into an 11-inch round. Lay each dough round in an 8-9-inch quiche pan and press dough to bottom and sides of pan so top is even with the top of the pan. Cover each dough pan with half of the cheese. Then divide vegetable ratatouille mixture in half and pour each half into dough lined pans. Beat the eggs with the cream, add salt and pepper to taste. Pour this mixture over ratatouille in each pan, while gently easing vegetables apart with a fork. Be careful not to puncture the dough. Let pans stand uncovered, until dough begins to rise, about 15 minutes. Bake pizzas in oven for 30-35 minutes, or until golden brown and fillings are set. Serve warm.

Approx. 255 calories per slice
8g protein, 12g fat, 30g carbohydrates,
33mg cholesterol, 432mg sodium, 3g fiber

PIZZA SAUCES

TRADITIONAL PIZZA SAUCE

Ingredients: Makes enough sauce for 15-inch pizza crust

3 cloves garlic, peeled and sliced
2 tablespoons extra-virgin olive oil
5 medium tomatoes seeded and chopped
2 sprigs fresh rosemary
Salt and pepper to taste
Pinch of sugar

In a heavy skillet over medium-high heat, Add oil and garlic, cook until it softens. Add tomatoes, herbs, salt and pepper, sugar, raise heat slightly and cook rapidly, stirring often until juices thicken, about 15-20 minutes. Put sauce through food mill, letting pulp go through. If sauce is too thin, return to low-heat and cook until desired consistency.

Approx. 63 calories per serving, based on a 2-inch slice
1g protein, 4g fat, 4g carbohydrates,
0 cholesterol, 390 mg sodium, 1g fiber

FIREY TOMATO AND BASIL PIZZA SAUCE

Ingredients: Makes enough for an 15-inch pizza crust

1 tablespoon extra-virgin olive oil
4 cloves of garlic chopped
5 medium tomatoes, seeded and chopped
3 tablespoons fresh chopped basil
Salt and pepper to taste
Pinch of sugar
1/4 teaspoon hot pepper flakes

In skillet, heat olive oil over medium-high heat, sauté garlic. Add tomatoes, cook and stir for about 5 minutes. Combine basil, salt and pepper, sugar, hot pepper and add to tomato mixture. Spoon the sauce onto desired pizza crust and bake.

> *Approx. 38 calories per serving, based on a 2-inch slice*
> *1g protein, 3g fat, 3g carbohydrates, 0 cholesterol, 7mg sodium, 1g fiber*

SPICY GARLIC OLIVE OIL AND SUNDRIED TOMATO PIZZA SAUCE

Ingredients: Makes enough for a 12-inch pizza crust

1/4 cup extra-virgin olive oil
4 cloves garlic, minced
6 jumbo pitted black olives, diced
8 sundried tomatoes in oil, drained and diced
1/4 teaspoon red hot pepper flakes
Salt and fresh ground pepper to taste

In a medium-sized skillet heat olive oil over medium-high heat, add garlic and sauté until translucent. Add hot pepper flakes, olives, and sundried tomato pieces, simmer over very low heat for 3-5 minutes. Spread over half baked crust; continue baking until crust is golden brown on edges.

> *Approx. 79 calories per slice, based on a 2-inch slice*
> *0 protein, 8g fat, 1g carbohydrates, 0 cholesterol, 42mg sodium, 0 fiber*

ANCHOVY AND GARLIC SAUCE (use for pizza or pasta)

Ingredients: Makes enough for a 12-14 inch pizza crust

6 tablespoons extra-virgin olive oil + oil from anchovies
6 cloves fresh garlic, pressed
2 oz. tin of anchovy fillets packed in oil, drained and chopped
Red hot pepper flakes to taste
2 tablespoons cilantro or parsley, finely chopped
6 tablespoons freshly grated Romano cheese
Salt and freshly ground pepper to taste

Combine oil and garlic in a skillet over medium heat and cook about 1-2 minutes. Add anchovies, cook about 30 seconds and remove from heat. Add in hot pepper flakes and cilantro or parsley. Add to pasta of choice or use as pizza sauce and serve. Add salt and pepper if needed.

> *Approx. 189 calories per serving, based on a 2-inch slice*
> *3g protein, 18g fat, 1g carbohydrates,*
> *13mg cholesterol, 387mg sodium, 0 fiber*

PIZZA CRUST

CRISPY THIN WHOLE WHEAT CRUST PIZZA DOUGH

Ingredients: Makes 15-inch crust (6-8 slices)

2/3 cups all-purpose unbleached flour
1 package active dry yeast
1/8 teaspoon salt
1/2 cup warm water
1 teaspoon extra-virgin olive oil
1/2 cup whole wheat flour
4 tablespoons all purpose flour
Non-stick cooking olive oil spray

In a medium mixing bowl combine all-purpose flour, yeast and salt. Add water and oil and beat on high speed for about 2-3 minutes. Use a wooden spoon to stir in whole wheat flour. Transfer mixture to a lightly floured surface and knead in 1-2 additional tablespoons of all-purpose flour as you bring mixture into a ball of slightly stiff dough consistency, yet still smooth and elastic. Put dough into a clean bowl, cover and place in a warm area for about 10 minutes. Spray a pizza pan lightly with oil spray. Roll out dough on a lightly floured surface to a 15-inch round, place on pizza pan and top with sauce of choice. Bake at 425 degrees for about 10 minutes, or until crust is crispy.

Approx. 76 calories per slice, crust only
2g protein, 0 fat, 16g carbohydrates, 0 cholesterol, 35mg sodium, 1g fiber

WHOLE WHEAT CRUST PIZZA DOUGH

Ingredients: Makes 15-inch crust (6-8 slices)

2 1/2 teaspoons active dry yeast
1 1/2 teaspoon Splenda or granulated sugar
1 teaspoon salt
2 tablespoons extra-virgin olive oil
1/2 cup lukewarm water
2 cups whole wheat flour
3-4 tablespoons of extra flour for kneading

In a bowl, mix together yeast, Splenda, salt, oil and water in a bowl. Set aside for 10 minutes. It will become cloudy and thick. When this happens, make a well in the center of the dough. Add yeast mixture and gradually fold in flour, adding more lukewarm water if needed. Knead dough until it becomes smooth. Place dough in a lightly oiled bowl and cover with clean cloth. Place dough in an area that is warm for about 45 minutes or until it doubles its size. Roll out dough on a lightly floured surface to a 15-inch round, place on pizza pan and top with sauce of choice. Bake at 500 degrees until crust is crispy.

> *Approx. 142 calories per slice, crust only*
> *5g protein, 3g fat, 22g carbohydrates, 0 cholesterol, 3mg sodium, 4g fiber*

THIN CRUST PIZZA DOUGH

Ingredients: makes 15-inch crust (6-8) slices

1 2/3 cups unbleached all-purpose flour
1/2 teaspoon salt
1 package dry active yeast
2 tablespoons extra-virgin olive oil
1/2 cup warm water
Olive oil to lightly coat pan

Put flour, salt and yeast in a large bowl and mix with a wooden spoon. Make a well in the center and add oil and water. Gradually work in flour from sides of the bowl as mixture becomes soft dough. The dough should be pliable and smooth. If too sticky, sprinkle a little more flour into mixture, but don't make dough dry. Transfer dough to a lightly floured surface and knead for about 10 minutes, add very small amounts of flour if needed until dough becomes smooth and elastic. Rub a small amount of oil over the surface of the dough and return it to a clean bowl, cover with a cloth and place bowl in a warm area for about 1 hour or until dough doubles in size. Remove dough to a lightly floured surface, knead for an additional 2 minutes then roll out to a 15-inch round, place on pizza pan and top with sauce of choice. Bake at 425 degrees until crust is crispy.

Approx: 115 calories per slice, crust only
2g protein, 6g fat, 18g carbohydrates, 0 cholesterol, 144mg sodium, 0 fiber

OMELETS OR FRITTATAS

CHEESY APPLE RAISIN CINNAMON OMELET
serve as a breakfast omelet or as a dessert

Ingredients: Makes 4 servings

1 medium sweet apple (figi, fugi or golden delicious), peeled, cored and sliced
1 tablespoon extra-virgin olive oil
2 tablespoons seedless black raisins
1 cup egg substitute or 3/4 cup egg whites or 4 whole eggs
2 tablespoons crumbled blue cheese
2 tablespoons freshly shredded Parmesan cheese
Salt and pepper to taste
1/8 teaspoon cinnamon

Sauté apples in 1/2 tablespoon of olive oil until crispy tender, add raisins. Remove apple mixture from pan. Combine eggs, cheeses, salt and pepper, mix well. Heat remaining oil in an omelet pan; cook 1/4 of egg mixture at a time, on low heat, lifting edges to allow uncooked portion to flow under and cook. Repeat process 4 times for each serving. Divide apple mixture into 4 portions and arrange each portion onto one half of each omelet. Fold omelet in half and sprinkle top of omelet with cinnamon.

Approx. 116 calories per omelet, using egg substitute
7g protein, 11g fat, 9g carbohydrates, 4mg cholesterol, 206mg sodium, 0 fiber

111 calories per omelet, using egg whites
6g protein, 11g fat, 8g carbohydrates, 4mg cholesterol, 166mg sodium, 0 fiber

166 calories, using fresh whole eggs
6g protein, 16g fat, 8g carbohydrates, 244mg cholesterol, 161mg sodium, 0 fiber

SPANISH OMELET

Ingredients: Makes 6 main course servings (often served as a light supper)

2 tablespoons extra-virgin olive oil
6 whole scallions, coarsely chopped
4 garlic cloves, thinly sliced
1 green bell pepper, seeded and thinly sliced
1 red bell pepper, seeded and thinly sliced
1 medium zucchini, diced
3 ripe tomatoes, peeled and cut into wedges
1/4 teaspoon cayenne pepper to taste
3/4 teaspoon ground cumin
1/2 teaspoon ground coriander
1/2 teaspoon ground cinnamon
Salt and freshly ground black pepper to taste
4 tablespoons fresh parsley, chopped
3 cups egg substitute or 2 1/4 cups egg whites or 12 large eggs
1/4 pound fresh goat cheese, crumbled

Preheat oven to 400 degrees F. Heat 2 tablespoons olive oil in an oven-proof skillet and gently sauté onions and garlic, for about 5 minutes, until they begin to soften. Add the green and red peppers, zucchini, and tomatoes, raise heat slightly and continue sautéing another 5-10 minutes until the vegetables have soften and most of the juice is absorbed. Add salt and pepper to taste. Set aside at room temperature. In a large bowl combine the herbs with the eggs, mix with a fork just enough to break up the yolks. Lift the vegetables out of the skillet with a slotted spoon and combine with eggs. Return the skillet to medium heat adding more oil if necessary.

(Continued)

When the oil is hot add the eggs and vegetable mixture and cook for 2-3 minutes, lifting the edges with a spatula allowing uncooked eggs to run under cooked ones. This starts the cooking process. Crumble cheese over the top of the omelet and transfer skillet to oven to finish cooking for about 15-20 minutes or until omelet is set and the cheese is melted.

Approx. 125 calories per serving, using egg substitute
10g protein, 13g fat, 6g carbohydrates,
8mg cholesterol, 190mg sodium, 1g fiber

121 calories per serving, using egg whites
9g protein, 13g fat, 5g carbohydrates,
8mg cholesterol, 150 mg sodium, 1g fiber

176 calories per serving, using fresh whole eggs
11g protein, 18g fat, 6g carbohydrates,
248mg cholesterol, 145mg sodium, 1g fiber

MIXED VEGETABLE FRITTATA

Ingredients: Makes 4 servings

10 large fresh asparagus spears
1 1/2 cups egg substitute or 1 1/8 cups egg whites or 6 whole eggs
3/4 cup low fat cottage cheese
2 teaspoons spicy brown mustard
1/4 teaspoon crushed dried tarragon
1/4 teaspoon marjoram
Salt and pepper to taste
1/2 teaspoon extra-virgin olive oil
1 cup sliced fresh mushrooms
1/2 cup diced onions
1/4 cup chopped seeded tomatoes for garnish

Preheat oven to 400 degrees. Boil asparagus for 8-10 minutes until crispy tender. Drain. Cut all but three spears into 1-inch pieces. Set aside. In a bowl, mix together egg substitute, cottage cheese, mustard, tarragon, marjoram, salt and pepper. Set aside. Heat olive oil in a large cast iron skillet, sauté mushrooms and onions until tender. Stir in asparagus pieces. Pour egg mixture over top, cook additional 5 minutes over low heat until it bubbles and begins to set. Arrange remaining three uncut asparagus on top of mixture. Bake uncovered at 400 degrees for 10 minutes or until frittata sets. Remove from heat. Sprinkle with tomatoes and serve.

(Continued)

Approx. 169 calories per serving, using egg substitute
17g protein, 9g fat, 7g carbohydrates,
321mg cholesterol, 369mg sodium, 2g fiber

164 calories per serving, using egg whites
16g protein, 9g fat, 6g carbohydrates, 321mg cholesterol,
329mg sodium, 2g fiber

216 calories per serving, using fresh whole eggs
18g protein, 14g fat, 7g carbohydrates,
561mg cholesterol, 324mg sodium, 2g fiber

BROCCOLI AND CHEESE FRITTATA

Ingredients: Makes 6 servings (often served as a light supper)

3 cups broccoli florets
1 tablespoon extra-virgin olive oil
1/2 cup onion, finely chopped
1/2 cup chopped red bell pepper
2 cloves garlic, minced
1 cup shredded mozzarella cheese
Dash of crushed red hot pepper flakes
1 1/2 cups egg substitute or 1 1/8 cups egg whites or 6 large eggs

Preheat oven to 325 degrees F. Steam broccoli until crisp-tender and remove from heat. In a large skillet over medium-high heat add olive oil, sauté onions, bell peppers and garlic until vegetables are soft, about 5 minutes. Add broccoli, cook about 2 minutes longer. Transfer vegetable mixture to a bowl, add cheese and crushed hot peppers. Beat eggs in a separate bowl until blended. Stir eggs into vegetable mixture and pour egg mixture into a greased round cake pan. Bake in oven until eggs are set, about 30 minutes. Serve hot or at room temperature.

> *Approx. 121 calories per serving, using egg substitute*
> *12g protein, 5g fat, 5g carbohydrates,*
> *10mg cholesterol, 209mg sodium, 0 fiber*
>
> *116 calories per serving, using egg whites*
> *11g protein, 5g fat, 4g carbohydrates,*
> *10mg cholesterol, 169mg sodium, 0 fiber)*
>
> *166 calories per serving, using fresh whole eggs*
> *12g protein, 9g fat, 5g carbohydrates,*
> *197mg cholesterol, 172mg sodium, 0 fiber*

ZUCCHINI FRITTATA

Ingredients: Makes 6 servings (often served as a light supper)

1 1/2 tablespoons extra-virgin olive oil
1 medium yellow onion, chopped
2 cloves garlic, minced
3 small zucchini, sliced 1/4-inch thick
Salt and freshly ground black pepper to taste
2 tablespoons minced fresh basil leaves
2 cups egg substitute or 1 1/2 cups egg whites or 8 large eggs
1/2 cup (2 oz.) freshly grated Parmesan cheese

Preheat oven to 325 degrees F. In a skillet over medium-low heat, add oil, sauté onions and garlic until soft and lightly browned. Add zucchini and salt and pepper to onion/garlic mixture and cook another 5-8 minutes. Remove from heat and set aside. In a bowl, add eggs (beat eggs if using whole eggs) to zucchini mixture, add basil. Stir mixture to blend and pour egg mixture into a lightly greased round cake pan. Bake in oven at 325 degrees until eggs set. Remove from oven, sprinkle cheese over top of frittata and place under broiler for 2-3 minutes until cheese is golden brown. Remove from oven and serve immediately.

Approx. 126 calories per serving, using egg substitute
12g protein, 6g fat, 11g carbohydrates,
7mg cholesterol, 312mg sodium, 1g fiber

121 calories per serving, using egg whites
11g protein, 6g fat, 4g carbohydrates,
7mg cholesterol, 244mg sodium, 1g fiber)

161 calories per serving, using whole eggs
10g protein, 10g fat, 4g carbohydrates,
195mg cholesterol, 242mg sodium, 1g fiber

VEGETABLE OMELET WITH PESTO

Ingredients: Makes 6 servings

1 recipe of pesto (page 268)
1/2 cup fresh peas, cooked and drained
2 whole carrots, cleaned, cut julienne style, cooked and drained
1/2 teaspoons extra-virgin olive oil
1 cup sliced white mushrooms
2/3 medium red onion, diced
Option- substitute other vegetables if so desired
Olive oil spray
3 cups egg substitute or 2 1/4 cups egg whites or 12 whole fresh eggs
1/4 cup water
1/4 teaspoon salt
1/4 teaspoon pepper
6 sprigs basil for garnish

In a medium skillet heat olive oil and sauté mushrooms and onions until tender crisp. Remove from heat. Mix all other vegetables with onions and mix in prepared pesto. Spray a non stick 15x10x1-inch baking pan with olive oil spray and set aside. In a mixing bowl, combine eggs or egg substitute with water, salt and pepper. Beat until frothy. Pour egg mixture into pan, bake uncovered at 400 degrees for about 8 minutes or until mixture is set. Cut baked eggs into six 5-inch squares and remove squares from pan. Spoon on 1/4 cup of vegetable mixture on half of each omelet square, fold over and garnish with basil spray.

Approx: 64 calories per serving, using egg substitute - without pesto
7g protein, 2g fat, 6g carbohydrates, 0 cholesterol, 137mg sodium, 2g fiber

59 calories per serving, using egg whites- without pesto
5g protein, 2g fat, 6g carbohydrates, 0 cholesterol, 97mg sodium, 2g fiber

114 calories per serving, using fresh whole eggs without pesto
protein, 7g fat, 6g carbohydrates, 0 cholesterol, 92mg sodium, 2g fiber

EGG WHITE AND ROASTED GARLIC OMELET

Ingredients: Makes 1 serving

1 jumbo roasted garlic clove or 3 small cloves, mashed
1/2 tablespoon extra-virgin olive oil
1/8 cup chopped red onion
6 tablespoons of liquid egg whites
Salt and fresh ground pepper to taste
1/4 cup diced fresh tomato
2 tablespoons shredded Parmesan cheese

Roast garlic in oven (left over roasted garlic works great). Set aside. Add 1/4 tablespoon olive oil to an omelet pan and lightly sauté onion. Remove onion from pan and set aside. Add balance of olive oil to pan and on high heat add egg whites, salt and pepper. As egg whites begin to solidify, lift edges of omelet around edge of pan and lower heat. Cook until omelet is solid. Add mashed garlic, red onions, tomatoes and cheese to 1/2 side of omelet. Flip other side of omelet over to cover mixture, cook until cheese starts to melt. Remove from heat and serve.

> *Approx. 160 calories per serving*
> *14g protein, 16g fat, 2g carbohydrates,*
> *12mg cholesterol, 250mg sodium, 0 fiber*

MAIN DISHES

SPANISH PAELLA WITH SAFFRON RICE, SEAFOOD AND CHICKEN

Ingredients: Makes 8 servings

12 medium size shrimp
7 hard-shelled clams
1/2 pound garlic- seasoned smoked pork sausage
2 lbs. chicken, cut into pieces, skin removed
Dash pepper
3/4 teaspoon garlic salt
1/2 cup extra-virgin olive oil
1/4 pound lean boneless pork, cut into 1/2-inch cubes
1/2 cup chopped onions
1/2 medium red bell pepper, seeded and sliced
1/2 medium yellow bell pepper, seeded and sliced
1 large tomato, peeled and finely chopped
2 cloves garlic, crushed
3 cups uncooked long grain rice
1/2 teaspoon salt
1/4 teaspoon ground saffron
6 cups water
1 cup frozen peas, thoroughly defrosted

Drain and rinse shrimp, place in a bowl off to side. Clean clams under running water, place on dish off to side. Prick sausage with fork in several places, place in heavy skillet, cover sausage with cold water. Bring water to a boil, and reduce heat to low. Simmer sausages uncovered for 15 minutes. Drain sausages well, slice into 1/4 inch round pieces and set aside. Rinse chicken, pat dry, season with garlic salt and pepper. Heat

(Continued)

1/2 cup olive oil in large skillet until very hot, add chicken pieces and fry until golden brown. Remove browned chicken from skillet and place on plate lined with paper towels. Add sausage pieces to skillet, quickly brown and drain on plate lined with paper towels. Remove oil from skillet and dry with paper towels. Add 1/4 cup fresh olive oil and heat until hot. Add pork cubes and brown quickly. Add onions, green peppers, tomatoes, and garlic. Cook vegetables and meat, stirring constantly, until most of the liquid evaporates. This is called Sofrito. Set aside. Preheat oven to 400 degrees F. In a large casserole, (14 inches wide by 2 inches deep) add the Sofrito, rice, and saffron. Bring 6 cups of water to a boil and add to skillet. Bring mixture to a boil, stirring constantly. Remove from heat and taste for seasonings. Arrange shrimp, clams, sausage, and chicken over rice, sprinkle peas over meats and seafood. Place pan on bottom rack of oven and bake for 25 to 30 minutes or until liquid is absorbed. Do not stir. When paella is cooked, remove from oven, cover with clean kitchen towel and let rest for 5 minutes. Serve immediately. Note, oven should be preheated one-half hour before paella is placed inside.

Approx. 523 calories per serving
38g protein, 13g fat, 61g carbohydrates,
117mg cholesterol, 819mg sodium, 3g fiber

SKEWERED MEDITERRANEAN GRILLED LAMB AND VEGETABLES

Ingredients: Makes 4 servings

1 1/2 lbs. lamb sirloin, cubed into 1 1/2 inch pieces, marinated overnight or for at least 8 hours
(marinate mix; juice from 2 lemons, 1/3 cup extra-virgin oil, 1 clove minced garlic, 1 tablespoon mint, salt and pepper)
8 large bay leaves
8 fresh mushroom caps
8 small cherry tomatoes
1 large green pepper, seeded and cut into 1 1/2 inch strips
2 small zucchini, cut into 1-inch cubes
4 medium onions, quartered
Salt and pepper to taste

Use 8 flat-bladed oiled skewers, alternate meat, bay leaves and vegetables on each skewer. Grill over hot coals about 15 minutes, turning skewers several times. This dish goes well with a chopped salad of onions, cucumbers, tomatoes, and parsley. Use lemon juice for a dressing.

> *Approx. 296 calories per serving*
> *38g protein, 8g fat, 15g carbohydrates,*
> *103mg cholesterol, 141mg sodium, 3g fiber*

BAKED STUFFED TROUT

Ingredients: Makes 4 servings

4 whole Trout (each about 12 oz.), scaled and gutted
3 tablespoons extra-virgin olive oil
1 large onion, finely chopped
4 cloves garlic, minced
2/3 cup plain breadcrumbs
1 lemon, juiced and rind grated
1/3 cup seedless dark raisins, chopped
1/2 cup pine nuts
2 tablespoons chopped fresh parsley
1 tablespoon chopped fresh dill
Salt and freshly ground black pepper to taste
1/4 cup egg substitute
Olive oil spray
Lemon wedges for garnish

Preheat oven to 375 degrees.   In a skillet heat 2 tablespoons of oil, add onions and garlic, cook until soften and remove from heat. In a large bowl mix breadcrumbs, grated lemon rind, raisins, pine nuts, parsley, dill and salt and pepper. Add garlic mixture, and egg and mix well together. Stuff each Trout with mixture and place in a single layer on a oil sprayed shallow baking pan. Make several diagonal slashes along the body of each fish and drizzle fish with lemon juice and remaining tablespoon of oil. Bake at 375 degrees for about 30-45 minutes or until fish flakes. Serve hot garnished with lemon wedges.

> *Approx. 579 calories per serving*
> *61g protein, 30g fat, 13g carbohydrates,*
> *284mg cholesterol, 547mg sodium, 1g fiber*

GREAT NORTHERN BEANS AND CHICKEN

Ingredients: Makes 6 servings

2 boneless chicken legs
2 boneless chicken breasts
2 cups reduced sodium chicken broth
2 onions, chopped into large pieces
5 carrots (1 sliced, others cut into large pieces)
2 stalks celery (1 sliced, other cut into large pieces)
4 cups canned Great Northern beans, drained and rinsed
2 tomatoes, peeled and chopped into large pieces
1/2 green bell pepper, chopped into large pieces
2 teaspoons fresh thyme
3 cloves fresh garlic, chopped
2 tablespoons fresh Parsley, chopped
Salt and freshly ground black pepper to taste

Remove all skin and excess fat from chicken. Rinse chicken under water and pat dry. Place chicken, half of the onion, 1 sliced carrot and 1 sliced celery stalk in a saucepan. Add water to cover chicken and cook over medium heat until chicken is tender. Strain and set aside. Preheat oven to 350 degrees. Grease a large casserole and add chicken, 2 cups of broth and beans. Cut remaining carrots and celery into large pieces and add to casserole along with tomatoes, remaining onion, green pepper, thyme, garlic, parsley and salt and pepper. Bake for 45 minutes until mixture simmers gently. Serve while hot.

> *Approx. 352 calories per serving*
> *34g protein, 7g fat, 39g carbohydrates,*
> *82mg cholesterol, 267 mg sodium, 2g fiber*

SPICY SOLE

Ingredients: Makes 4 servings

8 fillets of Sole, about 3 oz. each
1 cup water
1 cup dry white vermouth
1 tablespoon fresh lemon juice
Salt and freshly ground black pepper to taste
Top with a spicy pistachio pesto (page 273) (make sauce while fish is poaching)

Season fillets with salt and pepper and roll up, securing with a toothpicks. Set aside. Bring 1 cup water, vermouth and lemon juice to a simmer, add rolled fillets, cover and poach for about 7 minutes until flesh turns white and fish is cooked through. Add salt and pepper to taste and top with spicy pistachio pesto. Serve while hot.

Approx. 154 calories per 2 fillets
32g protein, 2g fat, 0 carbohydrates,
82mg cholesterol, 178mg sodium, 0 fiber

BOUILLABAISSE

Ingredients: Makes 4 servings

2 teaspoons extra-virgin olive oil
2 leeks, white and green parts, thinly sliced
3 cloves garlic, minced
2 cups freshly chopped tomatoes
1/4 cup dry white wine
1 tablespoon tomato paste
1 tablespoon freshly chopped parsley
1/2 teaspoon dried thyme
2 bay leaves
1/3 teaspoon crushed saffron
1/8 teaspoon fennel seeds
10 oz. fresh firm sole, cut into 1 1/2 inch chunks
Two (6 oz.) fresh lobster tails, quartered
16 littleneck clams, scrubbed
3 oz. Orzo, cooked and drained

In a large saucepan over medium-high heat, combine oil, leek and garlic, stir occasionally, and cook for about 3 minutes. Add tomatoes, 1 1/2 cups of water, wine, tomato paste, parsley, thyme, bay leaves, saffron and fennel seeds; stir to combine. Bring mixture to boil, stirring occasionally. Add sole, lobster and clams; return to boil. Reduce heat to low and simmer, covered for 6-8 minutes. Fish and lobster should be cooked until done and clams until they open. Remove bay leaf. Spoon cooked Orzo into 4 soup bowls; ladle Bouillabaisse over Orzo and serve.

> **Approx. 278 calories per serving**
> **29g protein, 4g fat, 26g carbohydrates,**
> **71mg cholesterol, 268mg sodium, 2g fiber**

SPICY BROCCOLI RABE WITH PENNE PASTA

Ingredients: Makes 4 servings

2 lbs. of fresh Broccoli Rabe, cleaned trimmed and cut into 1-inch pieces
1 lb. of whole wheat penne pasta
3 tablespoons extra-virgin olive oil
5 cloves garlic, thinly sliced
1 medium white onion, chopped
2 oz. anchovy fillets, drained
1/4 teaspoon crushed red hot pepper
Salt and freshly ground pepper to taste
Freshly grated Romano cheese for garnish (optional)

In a large saucepan bring water and salt to a boil. Add Broccoli Rabe and cook about 5 minutes until stems are tender. With a slotted spoon, transfer broccoli to a colander to drain. Return broccoli water to a boil and add pasta. Cook until tender and drain, reserving 1/4 cup of pasta water. Return pasta to a saucepan and keep warm. In a large skillet, heat oil, add garlic and onion, sauté for about 2 minutes until golden. Add anchovies and crushed red pepper stirring for about 1 minute. Add Broccoli Rabe and cook another 5 minutes until heated. To Broccoli Rabe mixture add pasta and enough of reserved pasta liquid to lightly moisten mixture, toss until well mixed. Add salt and pepper to taste. Garnish with Romano cheese. Serve warm.

> *Approx. 580 calories*
> *21g protein, 14g fat, 94g carbohydrates,*
> *8mg cholesterol, 645mg sodium, 7g fiber*

GRILLED CITRUS SALMON WITH GARLIC GREENS

Ingredients: Makes 4 servings

1/1 cup orange marmalade
2 tablespoons fresh lime juice
2 tablespoons fresh lemon juice
1/4 cup light soy sauce
3 teaspoons grated orange rind
4 (3 oz.) Salmon fillets
2 teaspoons extra-virgin olive oil
2 teaspoons minced garlic
2 (10 oz.) bags fresh spinach
Scant amount of olive oil to rub on fish
Salt and pepper to taste
1 teaspoon fresh garlic, mashed to rub on fish
1 heaping tablespoon capers
1 tablespoon balsamic vinegar
4 scallions, (2-3 inch lengths) thinly sliced (use mostly white and light green sections)

Whisk together marmalade, juices, soy sauce and orange rind; pour mixture over fillets and marinade for 30 minutes. Prepare grill or preheat broiler. Refrigerate while marinating. Heat olive oil in a heavy skillet over medium-high heat; add garlic and spinach, one bag at a time, sauté until wilted. Cook about 2 minutes, add salt to taste while stirring frequently. Turn heat to very low, to keep warm. Combine olive oil, salt and pepper, mashed garlic and capers. Rub mixture into both sides of salmon steaks. Grill the fish or broil 3-4 inches from flame for 2-2 1/2 minutes on each side. Set fish aside. Remove spinach from heat and toss with vinegar and divide equally on 4 plates. Add grilled Salmon fillet to bed of spinach on each plate and garnish with onions. Serve.

Approx. 250 calories
18g protein, 13 g fat, 14 g carbohydrates,
188mg cholesterol, 884mg sodium, 6g fiber

SICILIAN STYLE LINGUINE WITH EGGPLANT AND ROASTED PEPPERS

Ingredients: Makes 6 servings

2 large yellow peppers
1 small eggplant, peeled, cut into 1/2-inch cubes
2 tablespoons extra-virgin olive oil
2 tablespoons oregano, minced
2 tablespoons capers
4 teaspoons minced garlic
1 (35 oz.) can peeled plum tomatoes
1/2 teaspoon red hot pepper flakes
Salt and fresh pepper to taste
1 lb. linguine
1 cup fresh basil leaves, shredded
3/4 cup grated Romano cheese

Preheat broiler. Cut peppers in half and remove seeds. Cut each half into strips, place on baking sheet skin side up and broil until blackened. Set oven temperature to 400 degrees. Toss eggplant cubes with 1 tablespoon of oil. Place cubes in a single layer on a baking pan and bake about 25 minutes until very tender and browned, turning one time to bake evenly. Heat 1 tablespoon of oil in a large skillet over medium-high heat; add oregano, capers, garlic and sauté until garlic is lightly golden. Add eggplant, bell pepper, tomatoes and liquid, hot pepper flakes, salt and pepper to taste. Cover, reduce heat and simmer about 15 minutes-stirring occasionally. Cook pasta in boiling water, drain and return it to the pot. Pour sauce over pasta, add basil and gently toss. Sprinkle with cheese and serve.

Approx. 336 calories
13g protein, 10g fat, 50g carbohydrates,
15mg cholesterol, 461mg sodium, 6g fiber

PENNE WITH ROSEMARY AND BALSAMIC VINEGAR

Ingredients: Makes 4 servings

2 teaspoons extra virgin olive oil
2 cups zucchini, cut into 1/2-inch cubes
3-4 garlic cloves, minced
2 sprigs fresh rosemary, about 4-6-inches long
2 cups canned Italian peeled plum tomatoes, drained
1 tablespoon fresh oregano, chopped
Salt and pepper to taste
1 tablespoon balsamic vinegar
8 oz. penne pasta cooked and drained
1 tablespoon and 1 teaspoon fresh grated Parmesan cheese

In a large skillet, heat oil over medium-hot heat. Sauté zucchini, garlic and rosemary about 4-5 minutes. Add tomatoes, oregano and salt and pepper to taste. Decrease heat to a simmer and cook for about 10-12 minutes. Add vinegar and mix well. Place cooked pasta into a bowl, pour sauce over pasta and toss to mix. Sprinkle with Parmesan cheese and serve.

Approx. 231 calories
9g protein, 4g fat, 42g carbohydrates,
1mg cholesterol, 235mg sodium, 3g fiber

CHICKEN AND EGGPLANT

Ingredients: Makes 8 servings

2 medium eggplants, peeled and cut into 1 1/2 inch by 1 inch pieces
Salt and pepper to taste
1/2 cup extra-virgin olive oil
3 lbs. of Chicken divided into 8 servings
3 tablespoons extra-virgin olive oil
2 large onions, chopped
1 teaspoon of mixed spices—-to make mixed spices combine:
2 teaspoons allspice
1 teaspoon ground cinnamon
1 teaspoon ground cloves
1 teaspoon cilantro
1 teaspoon ground cumin
1/4 teaspoon freshly ground pepper
4 large tomatoes, peeled, seeded and chopped
2 teaspoons Pomegranate Molasses, (page 265)
3 tablespoons fresh squeezed lemon juice
Fresh ground pepper and salt to taste
2 tablespoons finely chopped parsley

To make Pomegranate Molasses: boil 3 cups of pomegranate juice over medium heat. Reduce heat and simmer uncovered, stir occasionally. Skim the froth until juice is reduced to 1 cup. Cool, bottle and refrigerate.

Salt eggplant pieces generously and let drain in a colander about 30 minutes. This rids eggplant of its bitter juices. After 30 minutes, rinse pieces under running cold water, squeeze pieces with hands to remove excess moisture and dry with paper towels. In a large heavy skillet; heat olive oil over medium heat. Add half of the eggplant pieces, sauté while

(Continued)

turning frequently until golden brown. With a slotted spoon; transfer pieces to paper towels to drain and soak up excess oil. Repeat procedure with remaining eggplant. Add more oil if necessary. Pour oil from skillet, allow to cool, wipe clean. Pat chicken pieces dry with paper towels. Place chicken in skillet with 1 tablespoon of oil and sauté, turning to brown evenly on all sides. Transfer pieces to plate. Pour off all but 3 tablespoons of drippings from skillet. Add onions and sauté over moderate heat, until golden brown. Add garlic and mixed spices, sauté, about 30 seconds while stirring. Add tomatoes, Pomegranate Molasses, lemon juice, black pepper, and salt to taste. Return chicken and any juices from plate to skillet, spooning tomato mixture around pieces. Bring to a boil and reduce to low. Cover and simmer about 45 minutes or until chicken is tender. Stir in sautéed eggplant and parsley, cover, and simmer additional 10 minutes. Adjust seasonings to taste. Serve with a side dish of pasta (optional).

Approx. 623 calories per serving
32g protein, 46g fat, 21g carbohydrates,
126mg cholesterol, 126mg sodium, 5g fiber

BROILED RED SNAPPER WITH GARLIC

Ingredients: Makes 4 servings

1 whole Red Snapper (about 2-2 1/2 lbs), scaled and gutted
3 tablespoons lemon juice
1 cup dry white wine
1 chili pepper, chopped
3 cloves garlic, finely chopped
2 tablespoons extra-virgin olive oil
Salt and pepper to taste
Olive oil spray
2 tablespoons chopped fresh oregano
2 tablespoons chopped fresh parsley
Lemon wedges

Marinate cleaned fish for 1 hour in the refrigerator in a shallow pan with 1 tablespoon lemon juice, wine; chili pepper and 1 clove chopped garlic. Preheat broiler. Whisk together; remaining lemon juice, oil, salt and pepper. Rub inside and outside of fish with mixture. Place fish on a oil sprayed broiler pan and sprinkle with oregano. Broil fish for about 10 minutes, basting often with oil mixture and turning once until golden brown. Meanwhile mix together remaining 2 cloves of chopped garlic and parsley. Sprinkle the parsley mixture on top of cooked fish and serve hot garnished with lemon wedges.

Approx. 185 calories per serving
25g protein, 8g fat, 0 carbohydrates,
46mg cholesterol, 81mg sodium, 0 fiber

PASTA WITH PINE NUTS AND SCALLOPS

Ingredients: Makes 4 servings

8 oz. Tagliatelle or Fettuccine
4 tablespoons extra-virgin olive oil
3 cloves garlic, finely chopped
1 leek, white part only thinly sliced
10 pitted black olives, halved
1/4 cup pine nuts
12 large sea scallops, halved
Salt and pepper to taste
2 tablespoons chopped fresh basil

Cook pasta in a large saucepan with boiling water until tender. Drain and return to saucepan, sprinkle with a small amount of oil to keep from sticking, cover and keep warm. While pasta is cooking, heat oil in a skillet, add garlic and leek, cook until soft but not brown. Add olives and pine nuts, sauté until pine nuts are lightly browned. Add scallops, cook until scallops are opaque. Add salt and pepper to taste. Add scallops and pan juices to pasta and toss. Sprinkle with basil.

Approx. 409 calories per serving
17g protein, 23g 41g carbohydrates,
45mg cholesterol, 139mg sodium, 1g fiber

SPICY SHRIMP WITH ANGEL HAIR PASTA

Ingredients: Makes 4 servings

1 1/2 lbs. medium shrimp, peeled and deveined
1 teaspoon Splenda Granulars or granulated sugar
1/4 teaspoon salt
1 tablespoon chili powder
1/2 teaspoon ground cumin
1/2 teaspoon ground coriander
1/2 teaspoon dried oregano
1 tablespoon and 1 teaspoon of extra-virgin olive oil
8 oz. Angel Hair pasta cooked and drained
Lime wedges

Sprinkle shrimp with sugar and salt. Combine chili powder, cumin, coriander and oregano. Lightly coat shrimp with spice mixture. Heat 1 tablespoon of olive oil in a large non-stick skillet over medium-high heat. Add 1/2 amount of shrimp and sauté about 4 minutes or until cooked. Remove cooked shrimp from pan and repeat procedure with 1 teaspoon olive oil and remaining shrimp and add sauce from pan. Divide cooked pasta into 4 servings, top with shrimp and garnish with lime wedges. Serve immediately.

> **Approx. 320 calories per serving**
> **28g protein, 4g fat, 28g carbohydrates,**
> **161mg cholesterol, 759mg sodium, 5g fiber**

FRUIT GLAZED SALMON WITH COUSCOUS

Ingredients: Makes 4 servings

1/2 cup of apricot jam
3 tablespoons thinly sliced green onion
2 tablespoons prepared horseradish
1 tablespoon white wine vinegar
1/2 teaspoon salt (divided)
4 (6 oz.) Salmon fillets- 1inch thick, skinned
1/4 teaspoon freshly ground black pepper
2 teaspoon extra-virgin olive oil
3/4 lbs. couscous
2 cups fat free chicken broth, heated

Preheat oven to 350 degrees. Combine apricot jam, onions, horseradish, vinegar and 1/4 teaspoon of salt, stir well with a whisk. Sprinkle Salmon fillets with 1/4 teaspoon of salt and pepper. Heat olive oil in a large non-stick skillet over medium-high heat. Add Salmon and cook for three minutes. Turn Salmon and brush with half of apricot mixture. Wrap skillet handle with foil and bake Salmon in skillet at 350 degrees for 5 minutes or until fish flakes. Remove from oven and brush Salmon with remaining apricot mixture. Serve each fillet with couscous.

To prepare couscous: Oil an oven proof dish and place couscous in dish. Pour in chicken broth and let sit for 10 minutes until couscous is tender and liquid is absorbed. Cover dish and keep warm in a low temperature oven until ready to serve.

> *Approx. 396 calories per salmon fillet*
> *34g protein, 18g   25g carbohydrates,*
> *94mg cholesterol, 344mg sodium, 0 fiber*
>
> *Approx. 198 calories per serving couscous*
> *7g protein, 0 fat, 40g carbohydrates,*
> *0 cholesterol, 184mg sodium, 2g fiber*

PASTA PRIMAVERA WITH SHRIMP

Ingredients: Makes 4 servings

1/2 cup fat free chicken broth
1 tablespoon + 1 teaspoon extra-virgin olive oil
2 dozen medium shrimp, cleaned, peeled and deveined
1 1/2 cups broccoli florets
1 medium red bell pepper, thinly sliced
1 cup halved button mushrooms
1 cup frozen peas
1/2 cup sliced scallions
4 cloves fresh garlic, minced
1 oz. (2 tablespoons) dry white wine
1 pound whole wheat penne pasta, cooked and drained
2 tablespoons freshly grated Parmesan cheese

In a large nonstick skillet, heat 1/4 cup broth, 2 teaspoons of olive oil and shrimp; cook until shrimp are pink. With a slotted spoon remove shrimp, set aside. To skillet add remaining 1/4 cup of broth, broccoli, pepper, mushrooms, peas, scallions and garlic. Cook, stirring frequently, 4-5 minutes, until vegetables are tender and liquid mostly absorbed. Stir in wine and simmer roughly 1 minute longer and add shrimp to vegetable mixture. Place penne pasta in a large serving bowl and toss with remaining olive oil. Add vegetable mixture; toss to mix well. Sprinkle with Parmesan cheese.

Approx. 526 calories per serving
24g protein, 8g fat, 78g carbohydrates,
34mg cholesterol, 218mg sodium, 12g fiber

TURKISH MUSSEL STEW

Ingredients: Makes 6-8 servings (serve with crusty bread)

6 dozen mussels, scrubbed and debearded
1 cup dry white wine
1 cup of water
1 medium onions, peeled and sliced
1 leek, sliced, white part only
6 cloves garlic, peeled
1/4 cup extra-virgin olive oil
4 large tomatoes, peeled and diced
2 large white potatoes, peeled, sliced about 1/4-inch thick
2 medium carrots, cleaned and chunked
1 pinch saffron
2 bay leaves
Salt and fresh pepper to taste
1/4 cup finely chopped flat leaf parsley

Clean mussels under running water, discard any that are gaping. In a large heavy sauce pan- add wine, water and mussels. Cover pan and steam mussels until they open (roughly about 7-10 minutes). Remove mussels from liquid and discard any which have not opened. Set mussel liquid aside. Remove mussels from shells and add a small amount of liquid to keep them moist. Strain remaining mussel liquid through cheese cloth and set aside. In a clean sauce pan gently sauté onion, leek and garlic until tender and add tomatoes and cook for a few minutes (1 or 2). Add potato slices and carrots, saffron, bay leaves and strained mussel liquid; cover pan and cook over medium-low heat until vegetables are tender (about 30 minutes). Add mussels to mixture and continue cooking until all is heated thoroughly, add salt and pepper to taste- remove from heat and stir in parsley. Serve while hot.

> *Approx. 236 calories per serving*
> *14g protein, 9g fat, 20g carbohydrates,*
> *28mg cholesterol, 297mg sodium, 1g fiber*

SPICY WHOLE WHEAT CAPELLINI WITH GARLIC

Ingredients: Makes 4 servings

1/4 pound whole wheat capellini
1/4 cup extra-virgin olive oil
4 cloves garlic, chopped
1 teaspoon diced hot peppers
Salt and fresh ground pepper to taste
Grated Pecorino or Parmesan cheese (optional)

Bring salted water to boil in a large pot. Add pasta and cook until al dente (about 8-10 minutes). In a heavy skillet over medium heat, heat olive oil and sauté garlic and hot pepper until tender (about 1-2 minutes). Drain pasta, toss with garlic olive oil mixture and mix well. Add salt and pepper to taste and sprinkle with grated cheese if desired.

> *Approx. 434calories per serving*
> *12g protein, 17g fat, 59g carbohydrates,*
> *53mg cholesterol, 46mg sodium, 2g fiber*

PESTO STUFFED SHELLS

Ingredients: Makes 4 servings

1 tablespoon extra-virgin olive oil
2 cloves garlic, finely minced
1 cup thinly sliced button mushrooms
1/4 teaspoon thyme
1 cup red bell pepper, diced
1/2 cup yellow summer squash, diced
1 can (15 oz.) chick-peas, rinsed and drained
1/2 cup sliced leek, white and green parts
1 cup part-skim ricotta cheese
Basil Pesto sauce (page 267)
3 oz. jumbo pasta shells, cooked and drained (about 12 shells)
Grated Parmesan cheese to taste for garnish if desired

Heat olive oil in a large skillet over medium-high heat. Add garlic, mushrooms and thyme and sauté about 6 minutes. Add bell pepper and squash, cook mixture until vegetables are tender-crisp. Remove from heat; stir in chick-peas and leek. Add ricotta cheese and 1/3 cup of pesto sauce and gently stir mixture. Spoon mixture evenly into cooked shells and garnish with grated Parmesan cheese if desired.

Approx. 404 calories per serving
14g protein, 22g fat, 39g carbohydrates,
23mg cholesterol, 356mg sodium, 5g fiber

GRILLED or BROILED SWORDFISH

(Goes well with a small serving of Ratatouille as a main course or a side dish of flavored rice or couscous)

Ingredients: Makes 4 (6 oz.) servings

4 (6 oz.) Swordfish steaks, each 1/2-inch thick
1 tablespoon extra-virgin olive oil to rub into steaks
1 1/2 teaspoons extra-virgin olive oil
Salt and freshly ground pepper to taste
6 teaspoons minced garlic
2 tablespoons capers
6 tablespoons fresh lemon juice

Prepare grill or preheat broiler. Rinse steaks under fresh water and pat dry. Rub both sides of steaks with oil and lightly sprinkle with salt and pepper. Mash garlic and capers together to form a paste, add lemon juice and remaining 1 1/2 teaspoon olive oil, salt and pepper to taste. Mix together well and set aside. Grill fish or broil for 2-3 minutes on each side. Be sure not to over cook or fish will be dry. Remove from heat. Drizzle caper/garlic mixture over each steak. Serve.

Approx. 230 calories per steak
28g protein, 10g fat, 2g carbohydrates,
55mg cholesterol,   265mg sodium, 0 fiber

STEAMED SEA BASS

(Serve with rice, vegetable and or couscous)

Ingredients: Makes 6 servings

**2 lbs. Sea Bass (try also Grouper or Swordfish) 1-inch thick whole fillet
if possible
2 1/2 tablespoons extra-virgin olive oil
8 thin slices red onion
2 cloves garlic, thinly sliced
10 medium dill sprigs
8 slices lemon, 1/2-inch thick
1 tablespoon capers, rinsed and drained
Fresh cracked pepper to taste
2 tablespoons dry white wine
Sea salt to taste
Parchment paper**

Preheat oven to 400 degrees. Cut parchment paper twice the size of fish and place on a baking sheet. Center fish on paper and drizzle with olive oil. Scatter onion slices, garlic and dill sprigs on top of fish. Add capers and sprinkle with cracked pepper and a splashes of wine. Wrap parchment paper around fish, folding top and tucking ends under fish to form a seal so steam cannot escape while baking. Bake for 30 minutes. Check after 20 minutes for doneness. Fish should be opaque in the center, if not rewrap tightly and continue baking for an additional 10 minutes. To serve, place fish still wrapped in parchment on a platter. Open parchment when ready to serve, sprinkle on salt and serve immediately.

> *Approx. 205 calories per serving*
> *28g protein, 7g fat, 4g carbohydrates*
> *62mg cholesterol, 103mg sodium, 0 fiber*

TAHINI BAKED FLOUNDER

Ingredients: Makes 4 servings (serve with fresh steamed vegetables and rice)

4 (3 oz.) fillets of fresh Flounder
2 tablespoons low-sodium soy sauce
2 tablespoons Tahini (sesame seed paste)
1/4 cup fresh lemon juice
2 tablespoons extra-virgin olive oil
Fresh ground pepper to taste
2 oranges, peeled and sliced

Preheat oven to 400 degrees. Place fish fillets in a baking pan. Whisk together soy sauce, Tahini, lemon juice, oil and pepper. Pour mixture over fish and top fish with orange slices, cover and bake for about 20-25 minutes or until fish flakes.

> *Approx. 377 calories per serving*
> *24g protein, 30g fat, 3g carbohydrates,*
> *41mg cholesterol, 69mg sodium, 0 fiber*

SPICY CHICKEN WITH COUSCOUS

Ingredients: Makes 4 servings

1/4 teaspoon ground cumin
1/4 teaspoon ground turmeric
1 teaspoon ground cayenne
1 pound skinless, boneless chicken breasts, cut into 1-inch strips
1 teaspoon extra-virgin olive oil
5 cloves garlic, finely minced
1(16 oz.) can fat free chicken broth
1 cup fresh peas
1 large white onion, diced
1 medium red bell pepper, diced
Salt and fresh ground pepper to taste
1 cup uncooked couscous
1/4 cup chopped fresh cilantro, for garnish

Combine cumin, turmeric and cayenne. Sprinkle evenly over chicken strips, set aside. In a nonstick skillet, add oil and heat over medium-high heat until hot. Add chicken and garlic, cook about 3 minutes until chicken lightly browned. Add broth, peas, onion and red pepper to skillet, bring to boil, reduce heat and simmer about 2-3 minutes until chicken is cooked through. Stir in couscous, cover and remove from heat. Let stand until liquid is absorbed. Garnish with cilantro.

Approx. 340 calories
34g protein, 4g fat, 38g carbohydrates,
66mg cholesterol, 746mg sodium, 3g fiber

CITRUS SCALLOPS AND SHRIMP

Ingredients: Makes 4 serving

3 cloves garlic, finely minced
2 1/2 tablespoons extra-virgin olive oil
1 1/2 lbs. fresh arugula
1/2 lbs. large sea scallops, cut in halves
12 large shrimp, peeled and deveined
4 oz. fresh orange juice
1/2 pink grapefruit, juice only
Juice from 1 lime
Juice from 1 lemon
1 teaspoon honey
1/2 teaspoon finely shredded orange zest
1/2 teaspoon finely shredded lime zest
1/4 tablespoon extra-virgin olive oil
Salt and freshly ground pepper to taste
2 scallions, sliced thin

In a large skillet over medium-high heat sauté garlic in 1 tablespoon of olive oil for 1 minute, do not burn. Add arugula, cover and cook 1 minute until arugula is wilted. In a separate skillet, over medium-high heat, heat remaining oil, add scallops and shrimp, cook until scallops are opaque and shrimp pink, gently turning to keep from burning. Transfer scallops and shrimp to a heated plate, cover to keep warm, set aside. Combine orange juice, grapefruit juice, lime juice, lemon juice, honey, orange and lime zest. Pour juice mixture into seafood sauté pan, return pan to medium heat.

(Continued)

Stir the bottom and sides of pan to loosen any browned bits, incorporating them into juices. Bring to a boil, cook until liquid is reduced to half amount. Add salt and pepper to taste, cook for a few seconds and remove from heat. Drain arugula, divide between 4 plates, mounding in center. Divide scallops and shrimp into four portions, arrange on top of arugula. Pour juice glaze over seafood and garnish with sliced scallions.

> *Approx. 309 calories per serving*
> *34g protein, 13g fat, 26g carbohydrates,*
> *45mg cholesterol, 276mg sodium, 2g fiber*

ITALIAN POACHED SCALLOPS

(Serve with risotto and or vegetables)

Ingredients: Makes 4 servings

1 cup fresh orange juice
1 pound fresh sea scallops
2 teaspoons grated orange peel
1 small ripe plum tomato, chopped
1 teaspoon chopped fresh marjoram
2 tablespoons sour cream
Fresh cracked pepper

In a nonstick large skillet over medium heat bring orange juice to a boil, reduce heat add scallops and orange peels. Cover and simmer 5 minutes or until scallops are opaque and tender. Remove scallops from heat and transfer to a plate, cover to keep warm. Add tomatoes and marjoram to orange juice sauce and simmer for roughly 2 minutes until liquid reduces to 1/2 of original amount. Stir in sour cream, cook until sauce thickens. Add salt and pepper to taste. Add scallops to skillet, mix with sauce and heat through. Serve immediately.

> *Approx. 148 calories per serving*
> *16g protein, 8g fat, 11g carbohydrates,*
> *34mg cholesterol, 380 mg sodium, 1g fiber*

GRILLED GROUPER

(Great with seasoned rice or couscous)

Ingredients: Makes 4 servings

1/2 cup ripe pitted Kalamata olives
1/4 cup plain bread crumbs
1 tablespoon capers, rinsed and drained
1 teaspoon extra-virgin olive oil
1 teaspoon lemon juice
1 clove garlic
4 (4 oz. each) Grouper fillets

Heat grill; place oil rubbed grill rack on grill over medium-high heat. In a food processor, process olives, bread crumbs, capers, olive oil, lemon juice and garlic until smooth. Set aside. Place fillets on oiled rack and grill uncovered for 5 minutes. Turn fillets over, brush with olive oil mixture and grill for additional 5 minutes or until fillets flake easily. Remove from grill place on platter and serve.

> *Approx. 159 calories per serving*
> *24g protein, 4g fat, 4g carbohydrates,*
> *45mg cholesterol, 388mg sodium, 0 fiber*

SPICY STUFFED TILAPIA

Ingredients: Makes 4 servings

4 Tilapia fillets, about 3 oz. each
2 cups prepared crab meat stuffing mix (1/4 cup per fillet)
3 oz. fresh spinach leaves, rinsed and drained
1 tablespoon extra-virgin olive oil
1/2 teaspoon fresh crushed garlic
Sea salt and freshly ground pepper
1/4 cup crushed dry roasted pistachios
Red hot pepper sauce to drizzle

Preheat oven to 350 degrees. Rinse Tilapia fillets under cold water and pat dry. Divide stuffing mix between 4 fillets; placing mix down center of each fillet. Fold fillets over and secure with wooden skewer. Spread spinach on a baking sheet. Place stuffed fillets on bed of spinach. Drizzle olive oil over fillets, scatter garlic evenly over fillets, and season with sea salt and fresh ground pepper. Scatter pistachios evenly over fillets and drizzle red hot pepper sauce over top. Bake at 350 degrees for 20- 30 minutes or until fish flakes easily. Serve immediately.

> *Approx. 240 calories per serving*
> *18g protein, 13g fat, 9g carbohydrates,*
> *47mg cholesterol, 59mg sodium, 1g fiber*

BAKED TILAPIA

Ingredients: Makes 2 servings

4 Tilapia fillets, about 3 oz. each
2 tablespoons extra-virgin olive oil
3 cloves garlic, minced
2 scallions, chopped, both white and green parts
1/2 cup fresh chopped parsley
Salt and freshly ground pepper to taste
Fresh spinach and halved grape tomatoes for garnish
Juice from 2 lemons
1 lemon, quartered

Preheat oven to 350 degrees. Rinse fillets under cold water and pat dry. Place fillets in a baking dish. In mixing bowl combine oil, garlic, scallions and parsley, pour over fish, cover and refrigerate for 30 minutes. Sprinkle with salt and pepper and bake at 350 degrees for 15 minutes or until fish flakes easily. Divide cleaned spinach on 2 plates. Remove fish from oven, place 2 fillets on top of a bed of spinach on each plate. Squeeze juice from 2 lemons over fillets and garnish with lemon wedge and serve.

Approx. 138 calories per fillet
15g protein, 5g fat, 3g carbohydrates,
43mg cholesterol, 46mg sodium, 0 fiber

GRILLED SWORDFISH WITH KALAMATA OLIVES

Ingredients: Makes 4 servings

8 Swordfish fillets (about 3 oz. per fillets)
Salt to taste
Fresh cracked pepper to taste
2 tablespoons extra-virgin olive oil
4 medium ripe tomatoes, seeded and diced
20 large pitted Kalamata olives, chopped
1 teaspoon chopped oregano
1 teaspoon chopped thyme
1 teaspoon chopped marjoram
Parsley sprigs for garnish

Season the fish with salt and pepper and brush with olive oil. Grill fillets over high-heat, 3 minutes each side. In a large skillet over medium-heat warm olive oil, add tomatoes, olives and herbs. Sauté for about 2 minutes, lower heat to low and cook another 4 minutes. Divide tomato mixture between four plates, place two Swordfish fillets on each plate and garnish with parsley.

Approx. 322 calories per serving
35g protein, 16g fat, 7g carbohydrates,
66mg cholesterol, 26mg sodium, 1g fiber

SPICY RIGATONI WITH MUSSELS

Ingredients: Makes 6 servings

1 lb. Rigatoni
Pinch salt
1/2 cup dry white wine
2 lbs. mussels, scrubbed and debearded
2 tablespoons extra-virgin olive oil
2 cloves garlic, minced
1 1/2 cups cherry tomatoes, halved
1 teaspoon diced hot red peppers (as desired)
Salt and freshly ground pepper to taste
10-12 arugula leaves, chopped

Bring water to a boil, add salt and pasta. Cook pasta until al dente. Remove from heat. In another pot over high heat, add wine and mussels. Cook until mussels open. Discard any that do not open. Remove cooked mussels from liquid. Set aside. Sieve mussel liquid, reserve liquid only. Shell mussels except for 12 mussels (to be used for garnish). In large skillet heat oil, add garlic and sauté. Add tomatoes, hot pepper and sauté for a few minutes. Add shelled mussels, 3-4 teaspoons of mussel liquid and season mixture with salt to taste. Drain pasta and toss with garlic mussel mixture and chopped arugula leaves. Divide unshelled mussels equally and garnish each plate with a few unshelled mussels.

> *Approx. 454 calories per serving*
> *31g protein, 10g fat, 54g carbohydrates,*
> *44mg cholesterol, 463mg sodium, 8g fiber*

LINGUINE and MIXED SEAFOOD (Baby octopus, shrimp, calamari, mussels and bay scallops)

Ingredients: Makes 4-6 servings

8 oz. natural clam juice
2 cups good dry wine (Pinot Grigio or Chardonnay)
Pinch sea salt
1/4 lb. baby octopus, cleaned
1/4 lb. shrimp, deveined and peeled
1/4 lb. calamari, cleaned, cut into 1/4-inch rings
20 mussels, cleaned
1/4 lb. bay scallops
3 tablespoons extra-virgin olive oil
3-4 cloves minced garlic
1/4 teaspoon freshly chopped hot peppers
8 small ripe plum tomatoes, chopped into small chunks
Pinch of sugar
1/2 tablespoon fresh chopped parsley
1/2 tablespoon fresh chopped oregano
Salt and freshly ground black pepper to taste
1/2 lb. linguine, cooked al dente, drain
10-12 arugula leaves, chopped
10 pitted Kalamata black olives, halved

In a large deep skillet, add clam juice, wine and salt. Prepare octopus, shrimp, calamari, mussels and scallops add to skillet. Bring to boil, cover and reduce heat to simmer, stirring occasionally until calamari and squid are almost tender, reduce heat to very low. Shell all but 9-12 mussels, set these aside for garnish. In a separate skillet over medium heat add oil and garlic, sauté until golden brown. Add red hot peppers to garlic mixture reduce heat to simmer and cook for 1-2 additional minutes.

(Continued)

Add tomatoes, sugar, parsley, oregano, salt and pepper to taste and simmer another 3-4 minutes, cover to keep warm, set aside. In a pot of boiling water and a pinch of salt cook linguine until al dente, drain. Drain juices off of seafood and pass through sieve, keep strained liquid. Add 1 cup of strained liquid to seafood mixture. Divide pasta into 4 servings on separate plates, add equal portions of seafood to pasta and toss. Add chopped arugula, toss gently into linguine and seafood. Scatter black olives on each serving, place 3-4 mussels in shells on each plate as garnish and serve.

Approx. 375 calories per serving
21g protein, 4g fat, 34g carbohydrates,
98mg cholesterol, 235mg sodium, 2g fiber

LAMB AND BLACK OLIVES

Ingredients: Makes 4 servings (goes well with rice)

2 tablespoons extra-virgin olive oil
3 cloves garlic, crushed
1-2 sprigs fresh parsley
2 lbs. lean ground lamb
2 tomatoes, peeled, and chopped
1/2 teaspoon dried rosemary
12 pitted black olives, halved
1 cup dry white wine

Heat olive oil in a large skillet; add garlic and parsley, sauté until golden brown. Add lamb, stirring until browned. Add tomatoes, rosemary, olives and wine. Stir, cover and cook 3-5 minutes until cooked through.

> *Approx. 475 calories per serving*
> *47g protein, 15g fat, 6g carbohydrates,*
> *149mg cholesterol, 251mg sodium, 1g fiber*

RIGATONI AND GROUND LAMB

Ingredients: Makes 4-6 servings

Spicy garlicky pesto sauce (page 268)
1 lb. ground lean lamb
1 whole onion, minced
1/2 teaspoon dried hot red pepper flakes
1 1/2 cups frozen peas
2 tablespoons spicy garlicky pesto sauce
Salt and pepper to taste
1 lb. rigatoni pasta
2-3 tablespoons fresh chopped mint

Make pesto sauce, set aside. In a heavy bottomed sauce pan cook lamb, onions and red pepper flakes for about 8 minutes until lamb is cooked, stirring occasionally to break up meat. Add frozen peas and cook for another 2-4 minutes.   Add pesto sauce, salt and pepper to taste, mix well and set aside. Cook rigatoni in boiling water until al dente, drain pasta and toss with lamb pesto sauce. Garnish with fresh chopped mint.

Approx. 399 calories per serving
20g protein, 18g fat, 34g carbohydrates,
45mg cholesterol, 95mg sodium, 3g fiber

BOW TIE PASTA WITH EGGPLANT AND BLACK OLIVES

Ingredients: Makes 4-6 servings

1 lb. Bow Tie pasta
1 small eggplant, peeled and cut into 1-2-inch strips
Salt to taste
3 tablespoons extra-virgin olive oil
1 medium onion, chopped
Pinch of crushed red pepper flakes
1/2 teaspoon dried oregano
6 cloves garlic, minced
4 tablespoons freshly chopped basil
12 pitted black olives, Nicoise or Kalamata, chopped
4 oz. crumbled feta cheese
chopped parsley

Cook pasta until tender set aside. Salt eggplant strips and microwave to reduce water content in eggplant. Squeeze each piece and pat dry. Heat oil over medium heat and sauté onions, red pepper flakes for 1-2 minutes. Add eggplant, garlic and oregano and sauté until eggplant is lightly browned. Add basil and olives to mixture.   Drain pasta and toss with eggplant mixture. Serve garnished with feta cheese and chopped parsley.

> *Approx. 416 calories per serving*
> *15g protein, 13g fat, 54g carbohydrates,*
> *16mg cholesterol, 354mg sodium, 10g fiber*

PASTA WITH RED CLAM SAUCE

(Use thin long pasta like spaghetti, or angel hair)

Ingredients: Makes 4-6 servings (1 cup cooked (2 oz. dry) angel hair pasta per serving)

**8-12 oz. dry angel hair pasta
1 cup dry white wine
1/2 bottle clam juice
3 cloves fresh garlic, finely chopped
1/4 teaspoon dried basil
48 small hard shell clams
1/2 white onion, chopped
2 tablespoons extra- virgin olive oil
1 lb. whole tomatoes, peeled, seeded and chopped
1/4 teaspoon dried oregano
Salt and pepper to taste
1 teaspoon chopped parsley**

In a large pot of lightly salted boiling water cook pasta to desired consistency, drain and hold. In a large skillet, heat wine and 1/2 bottle clam juice, add 1 clove chopped garlic, basil and clams in their shells, cover and steam until shells open. Remove clams from liquid, strain liquid through strainer to remove grit, set liquid aside. Reserve 16 clams in their shells for garnish, remove remaining clams from shells and return them to strained liquid. Set aside reserved unshelled clams. In a separate skillet, heat oil, add onion, remaining garlic and sauté until golden. Add tomatoes, oregano, salt and pepper, to garlic mixture and cook for 8 minutes. Add shelled clams with cooking juices to tomato mixture and heat through for another 2-3 minutes, stirring to blend tastes. Pour clam sauce over pasta, toss and garnish with reserved unshelled clams and parsley.

*Approx. 349 calories per serving
21g protein, 2g fat, 50g carbohydrates-
37mg cholesterol, 298mg sodium, 2g fiber*

PASTA WITH CLAMS, WINE AND RED HOT PEPPERS

Ingredients: Makes 4-6 servings

8-12 oz. dried spaghetti
48 small hard shell clams
1 cup dry white wine
1/2 bottle clam juice
2 tablespoons extra-virgin olive oil
3 cloves fresh garlic, finely chopped
1 small hot chili pepper, minced
4 tablespoons fresh parsley, finely chopped
Salt and fresh ground pepper to taste

In a large pot of lightly salted boiling water cook pasta to desired consistency, drain and hold. In a large skillet, heat wine and 1/2 bottle clam juice, add clams in their shells, cover and steam until shells open. Remove clams from liquid, strain liquid through strainer to remove grit, set aside liquid. Reserve 16 clams in their shells for garnish, remove remaining clams from shells and return them to strained liquid. Set aside reserved unshelled clams. In a large skillet, heat oil, garlic, chilies and parsley, bring to a sizzle and add shelled clams with strained juice, salt and pepper to taste, stir and heat through. Pour sauce over pasta and toss. Garnish with reserved unshelled clams.

> *Approx. 329 calories per serving*
> *21g protein, 2g fat, 48g carbohydrates,*
> *37mg cholesterol, 298mg sodium, 0 fiber*

WHOLE WHEAT SPAGHETTI WITH ANCHOVY AND GARLIC SAUCE

Ingredients: Makes 4-6 servings (1 cup cooked (2 oz. dry) whole wheat spaghetti)

8-12 oz. dry whole wheat spaghetti
6 tablespoons extra-virgin olive oil + oil from Anchovies
6 large cloves fresh garlic, pressed
2 oz. tin of anchovy fillets packed in oil, drained and chopped
Red hot pepper flakes to taste
2 tablespoons parsley, finely chopped
6 tablespoons freshly grated Romano cheese
Salt and freshly ground pepper to taste
Pitted black olives, and cilantro sprigs for garnish

In a large pot of boiling water add pasta and cook to desired consistency, drain and hold. Combine oil and garlic in a skillet over medium heat and cook about 1-2 minutes. Add anchovies, cook about 30 seconds and remove from heat. Add in hot pepper flakes and parsley. Serve over pasta garnish with grated Romano cheese. Add salt and pepper if needed. Garnish with black olives and sprig of cilantro if desired.

> *Approx. 443 calories per serving*
> *15g protein, 26g fat, 35g carbohydrates,*
> *18mg cholesterol, 552mg sodium, 6g fiber*

FETTUCCINE WITH SUNDRIED TOMATOES AND GOAT CHEESE

Ingredients: Makes 4-6 servings

8 oz. whole wheat fettuccine, cooked and drained
1/2 cup sundried tomatoes in olive oil, chopped
1 cup scallions, sliced
4 garlic cloves, minced
1 medium red bell pepper, thinly sliced
1/2 cup dry vermouth
1/4 cup fresh basil, chopped
10 pitted Kalamata olives
1 tablespoon capers, rinsed and drained
2 teaspoons oregano
6 oz. feta cheese, crumbled

Drain oil from tomatoes and reserve oil, set tomatoes aside. In a skillet, heat reserved tomato oil over medium heat. Add scallions and garlic to oil and sauté until lightly brown. Add red peppers and 1/4 cup of vermouth to garlic mixture. Cook peppers until tender crisp or until vermouth is almost evaporated. Reduce heat to simmer, add tomatoes, remaining 1/4 cup of vermouth, basil, olives, capers and oregano. Simmer about 5-8 minutes.   Cook pasta to desired consistency (al dente would be best), drain. Place pasta in a large bowl and toss with goat cheese, until well blended. Add Tomato mixture and toss again until well mixed. Serve.

Approx. 438 calories per serving
19g protein, 5g fat, 67g carbohydrates,
0 cholesterol, 613mg sodium, 3g fiber

FLORENTINE ROASTED PORK

Ingredients: Makes 6-8 servings (serve with a variety of your favorite vegetables)

4 lb. loin pork
4 cloves garlic, sliced thin
1/2 teaspoon dried rosemary
4 cloves
5-6 tablespoons water
6-8 tablespoons of a hearty red wine (do not use a cooking wine)
Salt and pepper to taste

Preheat oven to 350 degrees. If the skin of the loin has not already been scored, cut lines into skin about 1/8-inch apart. Cut through the flesh to the bone on one side and insert the garlic slices and rosemary. Press the cloves into the scored skin of the loin and place loin into a roasting pan with water and wine. Sprinkle loin generously with salt and pepper and roast for 2-2 1/2 hours or until meat is very tender, but still moist; basting occasionally.

Approx. 422 calories per serving
57g protein, 19g fat, 0 carbohydrates,
167mg cholesterol, 140mg sodium, 0 fiber

CHICKEN WITH POMEGRANATE SAUCE

Ingredients: Makes 6 servings (serve with rice)

1/4 cup extra-virgin olive oil
4 lb. chicken, boned, trimmed of excess fat and cut into small pieces
2 teaspoons paprika
Salt and pepper to taste
4 cloves fresh garlic, minced
2 medium yellow onions, chopped
1/4 cup fresh parsley, chopped
1 small hot banana pepper, finely chopped
3 tablespoons pomegranate molasses (page 265)
3-4 cups, canned chunky tomatoes, with liquid

Wash chicken, remove fat and cut into small pieces. Sprinkle with paprika, salt and pepper.   Heat oil in a saucepan, add chicken pieces and stir-fry for about 2-3 minutes, add garlic and stir-fry for another 2-3 minutes. Add onion, parsley, hot pepper, molasses and tomatoes; cover and bring to boil. Cook over medium-low heat for about 30 minutes until chicken is tender.

> *Approx. 753 calories per serving*
> *52g protein, 57g fat, 4g carbohydrates,*
> *224mg cholesterol, 365mg sodium, 0 fiber*

CHICKEN PICCATA

Ingredients: Makes 4 servings (serve with spinach linguine)

4 (3 oz. each) chicken breast fillets, lightly pounded
Salt and pepper to taste
2 teaspoons extra-virgin olive oil
3 cloves fresh garlic, minced
1 cup low-salt chicken broth
2 tablespoon dry white wine
4 teaspoons lemon juice
1 tablespoon all-purpose flour
2 tablespoons fresh parsley, chopped
1 tablespoon capers
Lemon wedges for garnish

Heat 1 teaspoon of olive oil in a large skillet, add chicken fillets and cook until fillets are lightly browned and centers cooked. Transfer chicken to a hot plate to keep warm. Add remaining teaspoon of oil and garlic to skillet and cook for 30 seconds to soften. Combine chicken broth, wine, lemon juice and flour in skillet where chicken was cooked. Stir to blend, continue stirring until mixture thickens. Stir in parsley and capers and spoon sauce over fillets.   Place each fillet on a plate, spoon mixture over fillets. Garnish with lemon wedges. Add hot cooked spinach linguine or pasta of choice.

> *Approx. 289 calories per serving with 1 cup of spinach linguine*
> *10g protein, 4g fat. 39g carbohydrates, 41mg cholesterol,*
> *68mg sodium, 1g fiber*

BROILED TUNA AND TOMATO

Ingredients: Makes 4 servings

4 (3 oz. each) tuna fillets
4 tablespoons extra-virgin olive oil
2 large cloves garlic, minced
1 tablespoon parsley
Salt to taste
Fresh ground pepper to taste
1 1/2 teaspoons white wine vinegar
8 (1/2-inch) slices fresh tomato
Italian parsley for garnish

Rinse fillets and pat dry, set aside. Combine in a covered container 2 tablespoons olive oil, garlic, parsley, salt and pepper. Add fillets, turn to coat well. Marinate fillets at room temperature for 2 hours. In another bowl, combine remaining oil, vinegar, salt and pepper. Arrange sliced tomatoes in a flat container in one layer and pour oil mixture over tomatoes, marinate at room temperature for 2 hours. Heat broiler, place tuna on grilling pan close to heat and broil each side of fillets for about 2-3 minutes. Arrange 2 slices of tomatoes on each plate; add tuna fillets to top of tomatoes and top tuna with parsley. Serve while hot.

> *Approx. 224 calories per serving*
> *20g protein, 32g fat, 2g carbohydrates,*
> *38mg cholesterol, 35mg sodium, 0 fiber*

SHRIMP IN SPICY BLACK BEAN SAUCE

Ingredients: Makes 4 servings (serve with rice)

2 cups canned black beans, rinsed and drained
2 jumbo cloves garlic, minced
3 tablespoons extra-virgin olive oil
3 teaspoons chili powder
3 teaspoons cumin
1 1/2 cups chicken broth
24 large shrimp, peeled and deveined
Salt and pepper to taste
Parsley, chopped for garnish

Sauté all but 2 teaspoons of garlic in 1 tablespoon of olive oil until almost browned. Add chili powder, and cumin, sauté for another minute. Add beans to garlic mixture, stirring frequently, cooking for another 3-4 minutes. Stir in chicken broth and transfer mixture to a food processor or blender. Puree mixture and return to skillet. Simmer sauce for 5 minutes, stirring often. Set aside. Heat 2 tablespoons of olive oil in a large skillet over moderate heat. Rinse and pat dry shrimp; season with salt and pepper. Heat oil and sauté shrimp with remaining garlic. Cook until lightly golden brown in color outside and cooked through, turning often. Remove shrimp from oil. Warm sauce and pour onto serving platter. Arrange shrimp on top of sauce and garnish with parsley. Serve immediately.

> *Approx. 216 calories per serving*
> *15g protein, 10g fat, 16g carbohydrates,*
> *13 mg cholesterol, 616mg sodium, 4g fiber*

LEMONY CHICKEN AND VEGETABLES

Ingredients: Makes 4 servings

3 tablespoons of juice from fresh lemon halves
1 tablespoon fresh grated lemon peel
2 tablespoons extra-virgin olive oil
1/2 teaspoon salt
1/4 teaspoon freshly ground pepper
4 cloves freshly crushed garlic
1 teaspoon paprika
1 1/2 lbs. skinless, boneless dark meat chicken
3/4 lbs. yellow squash, quartered lengthwise
3/4 lbs. zucchini, quartered lengthwise
1/4 cup chives, snipped in short lengths

Whisk together, lemon juice, peel, oil and salt and pepper. Reserve 2 tablespoons of mixture in a separate cup. Add to original mixture garlic and paprika and pour non-reserved mixture over chicken to marinade in a covered container in the refrigerator for 3-4 hours. When chicken is marinated; heat grill to medium-high heat. Remove chicken from marinade and place on grill along with squash, zucchini and juiced lemon halves. Close grill top and cook for 10-12 minutes or until juices from chicken run clear when pierced. Turn chicken 1 time while grilling. Cook squash; zucchini and lemon halves until tender and brown. Remove chicken from grill and cut into 1-inch wide pieces. Cut squash and zucchini pieces in half. Serve chicken and vegetables on a platter tossed with reserved marinade and sprinkled with chives. Garnish platter with grilled lemon halves.

Approx. 255 calories per serving
29g protein, 9g fat, 8g carbohydrates,
105mg cholesterol, 254mg sodium, 2g fiber

SIDE DISHES

SAFFRON RICE

(Use short grain rice such as Arborio)

Ingredients: makes 4 servings

4 cups low-sodium vegetable broth
1 tablespoon extra-virgin olive oil
4 tablespoons chopped shallots
2 cloves garlic, minced
1 cup Arborio rice
1 cup dry white wine
1/4 teaspoon crushed saffron threads
1/2 teaspoon dried thyme
Salt and pepper to taste

Bring broth to a boil, reduce heat to very low. In a large skillet heat olive oil, add shallot and garlic and sauté until soft about 5 minutes. Add rice and continue to sauté, stirring constantly to keep from burning. Add wine, saffron and thyme, stirring constantly, scraping in any brown bits from pan. When wine is absorbed, slowly add simmering broth, stirring constantly as broth is absorbed and rice has become tender (about 20-25 minutes). It's possible to have some of the broth left over. Add salt and pepper to taste.

Approx. 282 calories per serving
5g protein, 5g fat, 49g carbohydrates,
0 cholesterol, 87mg sodium, 2g fiber

ZESTY LEMON SWISS CHARD

Ingredients: Makes 4 servings

1 1/4 lbs. Swiss chard, cleaned and trimmed
2 tablespoons fresh lemon juice
1 1/2 teaspoons extra-virgin olive oil
1 tablespoon lemon pepper
Salt to taste
1/2 cup golden raisins
2 tablespoons pine nuts

Shred Swiss chard into thin strips and place in a large bowl. Combine lemon juice, olive oil, lemon pepper and salt; mix well with whisk. Drizzle lemon juice mixture over chard and toss. Add raisins, pine nuts and toss. Let stand for 15 minutes before serving.

Approx. 111 calories
4g protein, 4g fat, 20g carbohydrates,
0 cholesterol, 391 mg sodium, 3g fiber

ROASTED PEPPERS

Ingredients: Makes 4-6 servings

1 largo rod boll popporc
2 cloves garlic, peeled and sliced
4 tablespoons extra-virgin olive oil
Salt and freshly ground black pepper to taste

Clean peppers and pat dry. Place pepper on moderately hot grill or on a rack under a broiler, (1-2 inches from heat) turning often until skin is charred and blistered. Charring of entire skin takes about 15-20 minutes for this to happen. Remove from grill or broiler and place peppers aside to cool. Rub off blackened skins. Cut each pepper in half, remove stalk and seeds and cut into 1/2-inch strips. Place strips in a bowl, add garlic, oil, salt and pepper to taste. Toss and set aside for about 30 minutes before serving.

Approx. 116 calories per serving
1g protein, 9g fat, 7g carbohydrates,
0 cholesterol, 2mg sodium, 2g fiber

CLASSIC SPINACH AND PINE NUTS

Ingredients: Makes 4 servings

1/4 cup golden raisins
Boiling water to cover
4 tablespoons pine nuts
2 tablespoons extra-virgin olive oil
4 cloves garlic, chopped
1 1/2 bags (10 oz. bags) fresh spinach, cleaned
Salt and freshly ground pepper to taste
Fresh lemon juice and extra-virgin olive oil to taste

Place raisins in a bowl and cover with boiling water. Let stand for approximately 10 minutes until raisins are plump, drain well. In a skillet over medium heat toast pine nuts, stirring constantly for about 1-2 minutes. Remove from heat, set aside. In a large skillet, warm olive oil. Add garlic and sauté for 1-2 minutes until golden. Add spinach a little at a time until it all becomes wilted, stirring constantly, about 3-5 minutes. Pour raisins over spinach and mix well. With a slotted spoon, transfer spinach to a serving dish and sprinkle pine nuts over top. Serve immediately or if serving at room temperature add fresh lemon juice and extra-virgin oil to taste.

> *Approx. 112 calories*
> *5g protein, 5g fat, 14g carbohydrates,*
> *0 cholesterol, 89mg sodium, 3g fiber*

CHILLED STUFFED PASTA SHELLS

Ingredients: Makes 4 servings

1 cup (canned) hearts of palm, chopped and well drained
1 cup chopped zucchini
2 cloves fresh, finely minced garlic
8 large pitted black olives, chopped
2 tablespoons fresh parsley, chopped
2 tablespoons extra-virgin olive oil +2 teaspoons
4 teaspoons freshly squeezed lemon juice
1/2 teaspoon salt
1/4 teaspoons freshly ground black pepper
12 jumbo pasta shells, cooked al dente and drained
4 cups of mixed salad greens

Combine hearts of palm, zucchini, garlic olives and parsley in a large bowl. Whisk together olive oil, lemon juice, salt and pepper for vinaigrette. To bowl of vegetables add 2 tablespoons of vinaigrette, gently mix. Stuff shells with vegetable mixture, cover and refrigerate until well chilled. Refrigerate remaining vinaigrette. To serve; divide greens into 4 equal portions, top with 3 shells and drizzle with remaining vinaigrette.

> *Approx. 180 calories per serving*
> *4g protein, 10g fat, 21g carbohydrates,*
> *0 cholesterol, 281mg sodium, 2g fiber*

GREEK RICE

Ingredients: Makes 4 servings

1 cup short-grain rice
2 cups vegetable broth
1 tablespoon extra-virgin olive oil
2 teaspoons minced garlic
2 tablespoons finely chopped onions
5 oz. fresh spinach, cleaned and chopped
Salt and freshly ground black pepper to taste
1/4 teaspoon dried oregano
1/4 cup crumbled feta cheese
1 tablespoon lemon juice

Bring rice in vegetable broth to boil, cover tightly, reduce heat to simmer and cook until liquid is absorbed. While rice is cooking, heat oil over medium-high heat and sauté garlic and onion until golden. Reduce heat to medium; add spinach a little at a time to allow spinach to wilt while mixing in garlic. When spinach is wilted mix in salt and pepper to taste and oregano. Remove spinach mixture from heat add cooked rice, cheese and lemon juice; toss well.

Approx. 235 calories per serving
6g protein, 10g fat, 28g carbohydrates,
27mg cholesterol, 803mg sodium, 0 fiber

GARLIC RICE

Ingredients: Makes 4 servings

1/2 tablespoon extra-virgin olive oil
4 cloves fresh garlic, minced
1 cup Basmati long grain rice
2 cups fat free chicken broth
1/4 cup grated Parmesan cheese
2 tablespoons chopped fresh parsley
3 jumbo cloves roasted garlic, cut into small pieces
Salt and pepper to taste
Fresh chopped parsley or cilantro for garnish

In a skillet heat oil, sauté fresh garlic until golden brown. Bring rice in chicken broth to a boil, cover tightly, reduce heat to simmer and cook until liquid is absorbed. Remove rice from heat add oil and garlic, cheese, parsley, roasted garlic and salt and pepper to taste, toss well. Garnish with parsley and serve.

Approx. 165 calories per serving
6g protein, 4g fat, 28g carbohydrates,
5mg cholesterol, 178mg sodium, 0 fiber

COUSCOUS, TOMATOES AND BLACK BEANS

Ingredients: Makes 4 servings

1 1/2 cups vegetable broth
1 cup uncooked couscous
1 tablespoon extra-virgin olive oil
2 cloves garlic, minced
1/4 cup fresh lemon juice
1/4 teaspoon freshly ground black pepper
1 1/2 cups canned black beans, rinsed and drained
4 large plum tomatoes, chopped
1/2 cup red onion, finely chopped
Garnish with finely chopped fresh parsley

In a sauce pan, bring broth to a boil. Stir in couscous, remove from heat, cover and let stand until liquid is absorbed. In a small skillet, over medium heat add olive oil and garlic sauté until golden brown. Remove sauté pan from heat add lemon juice and pepper, mix ingredients through. Transfer couscous to a large serving bowl. Fluff grains with thumb and fingers to separate. Add in garlic mixture, black beans, tomatoes and chopped onions, stir gently to mix. Garnish with parsley and serve.

> *Approx. 289 calories per serving*
> *13g protein, 5g fat, 55g carbohydrates,*
> *0 cholesterol, 832mg sodium, 7g fiber*

BROCCOLI WITH FRESH GARLIC

Ingredients: Makes 4-6 servings

10-12 fresh broccoli spears, roughly 6-inches long
3 cups low-salt chicken broth
3 tablespoons extra-virgin olive oil
2-3 cloves fresh garlic, crushed
2 tablespoons chopped, fresh parsley
Salt to taste
Pinch of freshly ground black pepper

Cook spears in a large skillet of low-salt chicken broth until slightly undercooked (about 7 minutes). Test with a fork, do not overcook. Drain well and set aside. Heat oil in a large skillet over medium-high heat; add garlic sauté, until golden brown. Add broccoli, parsley, and seasoning to taste. Turn broccoli several times, mixing well with seasons, oil and garlic. Serve immediately.

Approx. 164 calories per serving
8g protein, 11g fat, 13g carbohydrates,
0 cholesterol, 63mg sodium, 7g fiber

CRISPY TENDER RATATOUILLE *(serve with crusty bread)*

Ingredients: Makes 8 servings

3/4 cups extra-virgin olive oil
2 large onions, chopped
8 garlic cloves, minced
4 large ripe tomatoes, cored and diced
4 small zucchini, cut to 1 1/2 inch cubes
2 large eggplant, rinsed and cut into 1 1/2 inch cubes
3 red bell peppers, roasted, peeled and cut into strips
1 cup dry red wine
1 tablespoon of capers, rinsed and drained
1 or 2 pinches crushed hot red pepper flakes or to taste
Salt and freshly ground black pepper to taste
Freshly chopped basil for garnish (optional)
Pitted black olives for garnish (optional)

Place eggplant cubes in a bowl and salt and water to cover. Place heavy plate inside bowl to weight down cubes submerging in brine. Set aside for 1 1/2 - 2 hours. Roast bell peppers under broiler in oven until skins turn black and are easy to remove. Peel off skins and cut peppers into long strips. Set aside. Heat 1/4 cup of olive oil in a large skillet over medium-low heat, add onions and garlic and cook until soft. Do not brown onions and garlic. Add roasted pepper to mixture. Drain eggplant cubes, pat dry with paper towels. Add another 1/4 cup olive oil to skillet, increase heat to medium and sauté eggplant cubes until golden brown, about 15 minutes. Remove from heat and add other vegetables.

(Continued)

Add zucchini to skillet and cook, adding more olive oil if needed. When zucchini is cooked, add tomatoes, lowering heat slightly, stir in wine and simmer until wine is evaporated and mixture turns to a jam consistency, about 20 minutes. Stir in capers and hot pepper flakes and combine all vegetables to tomatoes sauce. Using a slotted spoon stir to mix, but don't break up vegetables. Add salt and pepper to taste. Before serving, add basil and black olives if desired.

> **Approx. 218 calories**
> **4g protein, 17g fat, 31g carbohydrates,**
> **0 cholesterol, 182mg sodium, 9g fiber**

GARLICKY SWISS CHARD

Ingredients: Makes 6 servings or 3 cups

2 bunches Swiss chard (about 1 1/2 lbs. each) cleaned and trimmed
3 tablespoons extra-virgin olive oil
6 cloves fresh garlic, minced
1/2 cup chicken broth
1/4 teaspoon hot cherry peppers, finely minced
1/2 teaspoon salt
1/4 teaspoon freshly ground black pepper

Rinse greens well and cut ribs and stems into 2-inch pieces. Set aside. Break leaves into roughly 2-inch pieces. Heat oil in a large heavy bottom skillet; add garlic and sauté until golden brown, stirring constantly. Add chard ribs and stems, broth and hot peppers, cook until almost tender. Add leaves in bunches, stirring to wilt. Stir in salt, pepper. Cook covered, until tender and liquid is evaporated, stirring often.

Approx. 100 calories per serving
4g protein, 7g fat, 8g carbohydrates,
0 cholesterol, 615mg sodium, 3g fiber

ORZO WITH FETA CHEESE AND BROCCOLI FLORETS

Ingredients: Makes 8 servings

2 cups broccoli florets
3 cups low-salt chicken broth
8 oz. uncooked Orzo (about 1 cup)
6 oz. feta cheese

In boiling water, cook broccoli florets until crispy tender. Drain, set aside and keep warm. In a saucepan bring chicken broth to a boil, reduce heat, add Orzo and cook until liquid is absorbed. Stir often to keep from burning. Fluff Orzo with fork and add feta cheese, stirring to blend together. Transfer Orzo to serving platter and top with broccoli florets.

Approx. 180 calories per serving
8g protein, 7g fat, 23g carbohydrates,
21mg cholesterol, 293mg sodium, 1g fiber

LEMON GARLIC ASPARAGUS

Ingredients: Makes 4-6 servings

1 lemon
1 cup shredded fresh Parmesan cheese
3 tablespoons extra-virgin olive oil
1 clove fresh garlic, crushed
2 lbs. fresh asparagus, cleaned, ends trimmed
Salt and coarsely ground black pepper to taste
2 tablespoons sweet orange juice

Grate lemon to make 3/4 teaspoon of peel. Using a vegetable peeler remove enough shavings from wedge of cheese to equal 1 cup of loosely packed cheese. Set aside. In a nonstick large skillet, heat oil over medium heat until hot. Add asparagus, garlic, salt and pepper; turn several times to coat asparagus with oil. Cover skillet and cook for 6-7 minutes or until asparagus is tender and lightly browned. Remove from heat. Sprinkle with orange juice and lemon peel. Transfer to serving platter and top with Parmesan shavings.

> *Approx. 115 calories per serving*
> *5g protein, 10g fat, 1g carbohydrates,*
> *7mg cholesterol, 475mg sodium, 1g fiber*

FAVA BEANS WITH PESTO SAUCE

Ingredients: Makes 6 servings (side dish or great for a quick lunch)

Spicy Garlicky Pesto Sauce (page 268)
3 cans (15 oz. each) cooked Fava beans, rinsed and drained
6 large lettuce leaves
1 small red onion, chopped
1/2 red bell pepper, diced
1/2 yellow pepper, diced
Salt and pepper to taste
Tomato wedges for garnish

Make pesto sauce, set aside. In a small bowl, mix pesto sauce with Fava beans. Arrange lettuce on platter or on individual plates. Pile pesto bean mixture on top of lettuce. Scatter onion and diced peppers over bean mixture. Add salt and pepper to taste and garnish with tomato wedges.

> *Approx. 162 calories per serving*
> *8g protein, 6g fat, 19g carbohydrates,*
> *2mg cholesterol, 621mg sodium, 5g fiber*

FETA AND MIXED BEANS

Ingredients: Makes 4 servings (side dish or great for a quick lunch)

1 (16 oz.) can white Kidney beans, rinsed and drained
1 (16 oz.) can Cannellini beans, rinsed and drained
1 (16 oz.) can chickpeas, rinsed and drained
3 oz. fresh feta cheese, crumbled
1 cup finely chopped red onion
3 tablespoons chopped fresh mint
1 1/2 tablespoon Splenda or granulated cane sugar if desired
2 cloves fresh garlic, finely chopped
1/4 teaspoon salt
1/4 teaspoon freshly ground black pepper
2 tablespoons + 1 teaspoon fresh squeezed lemon juice
1 tablespoon balsamic vinegar
1 teaspoon extra-virgin olive oil
4 cups mixed greens

Combine beans, cheese, onion and mint, stir and add Splenda, stir to mix well. Add to bean mixture garlic, salt and pepper, lemon juice, vinegar and olive oil. Toss again. Place 1 cup of greens on each plate, divide bean mixture into four servings and top each plate of greens with bean mixture and serve.

> *Approx. 230 calories per serving*
> *13g protein, 6g fat, 29g carbohydrates,*
> *20mg cholesterol, 660mg sodium, 6g fiber*

TUSCAN BRAISED FENNEL

Ingredients: Makes 4 servings

4 fennel bulbs
4 tablespoons extra-virgin olive oil
2 cloves garlic, peeled and sliced
Salt and coarsely ground pepper to taste
2 cups vegetable broth
Garnish with grated Parmesan cheese

Wash and trim bulbs. Cut tops off bulbs and reserve for garnish. Pat dry bulbs and cut into quarters. Place pieces of fennel flat side down in heavy skillet together with oil, garlic and seasonings. Cook over moderate heat, turning, until fennel pieces are browned. Add broth, bring to a boil, cover and reduce heat to low-simmer. Cook another 30-40 minutes until fennel is tender and liquid is absorbed. Sprinkle with cheese and serve.

> *Approx. 213 calories per serving*
> *4g protein, 14g fat, 7g carbohydrates,*
> *0 cholesterol, 295mg sodium, 3g fiber*

CHICKPEAS WITH COUSCOUS

Ingredients: Makes 4 servings (serve as side dish or with toasted pita bread as a quick lunch)

1 1/2 cups fat free chicken broth
1/3 cup couscous, uncooked
1 (15 oz.) can chickpeas, rinsed and drained
1 medium tomato, chopped
1/4 cup pitted sliced kalamata olives
1 stalk celery, finely chopped
2 large scallions, green and white parts, sliced into 1-inch pieces
1/4 cup black seedless raisins
1/2 teaspoon cumin
1/4 cup non-fat plain yogurt
Chopped fresh parsley, optional

Bring chicken broth to a boil, remove from heat and add couscous. Cover and let stand until couscous is tender and liquid is absorbed. Fluff with a fork and turn into a bowl. Add chickpeas, tomato, olives, celery, scallions, raisins and cumin. Stir to mix well and garnish with 1 tablespoon of yogurt and parsley.

> *Approx. 380 calories per serving*
> *12g protein, 5g fat, 71g carbohydrates,*
> *0 cholesterol, 453mg sodium, 10g fiber*

SPICY COUSCOUS

Ingredients: Makes 4-6 servings

2 1/4 teaspoons extra virgin olive oil
4 cloves fresh garlic, minced
1 small onion, coarsely chopped
3 cups fat free vegetable broth or chicken broth
3 cups couscous
2 teaspoons of ground cayenne pepper to taste
1 teaspoon Harissa if desired (page 264)
   — add more or less according to degree of spiciness desired
Ground cilantro leaves to taste
Salt and freshly ground black pepper to taste

In a skillet, heat 1 teaspoon oil, add garlic and onion, sauté until golden. In a saucepan bring broth and remaining oil to a boil. Place couscous in oven proof dish and pour hot broth and garlic mixture over couscous, stir to mix. Let stand for 10 minutes until broth is absorbed. Fluff couscous between fingers and thumb to separate grains. Add cayenne, Harissa and cilantro to taste as you fluff couscous grains, add salt and pepper to taste. Cover tightly to keep warm. Sprinkle additional cayenne and cilantro on top just before serving.

Approx. 154 calories per serving
5g protein, 1g fat, 32g carbohydrates,
3mg cholesterol, 485mg sodium, 0 fiber

SAUTÉED VEGETABLES WITH FRESH THYME

Ingredients: Makes 4 servings

2 leeks
1 medium red bell pepper
2 medium celery stalks
2 small zucchini (6-8 oz.)
1 medium eggplant
4 tablespoons extra-virgin olive oil
Salt and freshly ground black pepper to taste
2 tablespoons minced fresh thyme
5 medium garlic cloves, minced
2 tablespoons minced fresh parsley

Clean sand from leeks. Cut 2-inch pieces of white and green parts of leek, flatten each piece and cut into 1/3-inch slices. Separate slices. Cut pepper in half and de-seed. Cut pepper into 2-inch strips. Peel strings from celery and cut into 2-inch pieces. Cut zucchini in half and then into pieces roughly 1/4 x 1/4-inch. Peel eggplant and cut into pieces (2-inch x 1/2-inch thick). In a large skillet heat 2 tablespoons of olive oil, sauté eggplant over medium heat. Sprinkle with salt, tossing constantly until crispy tender. Remove eggplant from skillet, set aside on a paper towel dressed platter, to absorbed excess oil from eggplant.

(Continued)

Place platter in heated oven to keep vegetable warm. Heat additional tablespoon of oil in eggplant skillet, add leeks cook about 5 minutes, stirring often. Add red pepper, celery, salt, pepper and thyme and continue cooking, tossing often until vegetables are crispy tender. With a slotted spoon, transfer mixture to eggplant platter. Add zucchini and additional tablespoon of oil if needed to skillet and cook zucchini until tender. Remove zucchini to eggplant platter. Add garlic to skillet and sauté for about 30 seconds, do not brown. Add parsley, heat additional 2-3 seconds. Transfer all vegetables from eggplant platter to a clean platter and pour garlic/parsley mixture over vegetables and toss, mixing well. Serve immediately.

> *Approx. 140 calories per serving*
> *3g protein, 14g fat, 22g carbohydrates,*
> *0 cholesterol, 36mg sodium, 6g fiber*

CINNAMON COUSCOUS

Ingredients: Makes 6-8 servings

3 cups couscous
3 cups warmed water
Pinch of salt
1/2 tablespoon extra-virgin olive oil
2 tablespoons ground cinnamon
1/4 cup black seedless raisins
1/4 cup Splenda (packets)
4 tablespoons Mazahar (orange blossom water)
Coarsely chopped walnuts for garnish

Bring liquid to a boil; add salt and oil. Place couscous in an oiled oven-proof dish. Pour liquid over couscous, add 1 tablespoon cinnamon, raisins, Splenda and orange blossom water, let stand for about 10 minutes or until liquid is absorbed. Fluff couscous with fingers to separate grains. When ready to serve, top couscous with remaining cinnamon and walnuts.

Approx. 155 calories per serving
5g protein, 1g fat, 31g carbohydrates,
0 cholesterol, 14mg sodium, 2g fiber

SWISS CHARD AND ARBORIO RICE

Ingredients: Makes 6 servings

5 cups fat free chicken broth
2 1/2 tablespoons extra-virgin olive oil
1 medium onion, chopped
1 3/4 cups Arborio rice
1 Bunch Swiss chard (about 10 leaves), spines cut to 1/4 -inch pieces, leaves coarsely chopped
1/2 teaspoon dried rosemary, crumbled
1/2 cup dry white wine
Salt and freshly ground black pepper to taste
1/2 cup freshly grated Parmesan cheese (reserve a small amount for garnish, if desired)

Bring broth to a simmer, cover set aside and keep moderately hot. In a heavy bottom skillet; heat oil and sauté onions until translucent. Add rice, chard and rosemary, stir until chard wilts. Add wine and simmer until liquid is absorbed. Add 4 1/2 cups of broth and simmer until rice is tender and creamy, stirring often. Add remaining 1/2 cup of broth slowly as needed if mixture appears too dry, cooking about 20 minutes. Add salt and pepper to taste and Parmesan cheese. Serve immediately, garnished with a small amount cheese if desired.

Approx. 378 calories per serving
12g protein, 9g fat, 60g carbohydrates,
5mg cholesterol, 686mg sodium, 2g fiber

BASIC RICE PILAF

Ingredients: Makes 6 servings

**3 cups fat free chicken broth
2 1/2 tablespoons extra-virgin olive oil
1/4 cups toasted pine nuts
1/4 cup chopped blanched almonds
1 medium onion, finely chopped
1 1/2 cup long grain rice, like Basmati rice
2 cups frozen peas
Salt and freshly ground black pepper to taste
Chopped fresh cilantro for garnish**

Heat chicken stock, slowly simmer. Place 2 tablespoons oil in a heavy bottomed skillet, gently sauté almonds and pine nuts, toast but do not burn. Remove nuts from heat with a slotted spoon and set aside. Add onions to oil sauté and cook until soft, do not brown. Add rice to oil, sauté over medium heat for 10-15 minutes, stirring all the while until rice is crispy. Pour in hot chicken broth, add peas, 1/2 teaspoon olive oil, salt and pepper to taste. Reduce heat, cover and simmer until liquid is absorbed, about 20 minutes, Remove from heat, cover and set aside for 5 minutes before serving. Garnish with chopped cilantro.

*Approx. 335 calories per serving
12g protein, 14g fat, 44g carbohydrates,
7 mg cholesterol, 307mg sodium, 5g fiber*

ROASTED GARLIC (great with crusty bread or pita wedges also great as topper on cooked vegetables and omelets)

Ingredients: Makes 4 servings

1 jumbo garlic (4-5 large cloves)
Seasoned garlic salt to taste
Extra- virgin olive oil to drizzle

Preheat oven to 400 degrees. Cut the point off of jumbo garlic cloves and remove loose leaves. Try to keep cloves intact. Place jumbo cloves in an oven safe dish, sprinkle with a small amount of garlic salt and drizzle with oil. Bake cloves at 400 degrees for 20-30 minutes or until cloves are soft and golden brown.

BAKED EGGPLANT WITH GARLIC AND BASIL

Ingredients: Makes 4-6 servings

2 medium Eggplant
4 fresh cloves garlic, finely chopped
4 tablespoons extra-virgin olive oil
1 1/2 teaspoons fresh basil, chopped
1 tablespoon tomato paste
Salt and pepper to taste
2 tablespoons freshly grated Parmesan cheese
Finely chopped fresh rosemary

Preheat oven to 350 degrees. Wash and dry eggplants. Cut each eggplant into half lengthwise. With a sharp knife make a crisscross pattern in the skin of each eggplant. Put eggplants on a lightly oiled baking sheet and set aside. Mix together garlic, oil, and basil and tomato paste. Spread mixture onto tops of eggplants and bake at 350 degrees for 45 minutes or until tender. Remove from oven and garnish with cheese and Rosemary.

> *Approx. 139 calories per serving*
> *3g protein, 10g fat, 12g carbohydrates,*
> *1mg cholesterol, 30mg sodium, 4g fiber*

POLENTA

Ingredients: Makes 4-6 servings (Often used as a substitute for potatoes, rice or pasta, especially in Northern Italy)

3 cups of boiling water
2 teaspoons salt
1 cup polenta
Extra-virgin olive oil if desired
Grated Parmesan cheese for garnish

Bring water to boil in a saucepan and add salt. Slowly add polenta, bring back to a boil, while stirring constantly. Lower heat to a simmer, stir frequently for roughly 20-25 minutes or until polenta thickens. Serve with a drizzle of olive oil and sprinkled with cheese.

Approx. 106 calories per 1/2 cup serving
3g protein, 2g fat,
18g carbohydrates, 0 cholesterol, 246mg sodium, 0 fiber

POLENTA WITH MUSHROOMS AND GARLIC

Ingredients: Makes 4-6 servings

1 tablespoon extra-virgin olive oil
3 large cloves garlic, minced
3 oz. white button mushroom, cleaned and sliced
2 sprigs thyme, cut off stalks
3 cups boiling water
1 cup polenta
Salt and freshly ground black pepper to taste

In a skillet heat oil and gently sauté garlic and mushrooms until soft. Add thyme, stir to blend and set aside. Bring water to a boil, add polenta, continue boiling for 2-3 minutes, reduce to a simmer and cook, stirring frequently for about 20-25 minutes, until polenta thickens and liquid is absorbed. Remove from heat, transfer to a bowl, stir in mushroom mixture, add salt and pepper to taste. Serve.

> *Approx: 130 calories per 1/2 cup serving*
> *3g protein, 5g fat, 18g carbohydrates,*
> *0 cholesterol, 246 mg sodium, 0 fiber*

GARLICKY CANNELLINI BEANS

Ingredients: Makes 4 servings

2 (15 oz.) cans cannellini beans
4-5 large fresh cloves garlic, minced
2 tablespoons extra-virgin olive oil
1/2 cup chicken broth
Salt and freshly ground black pepper to taste

Rinse and drain beans. Cook garlic and oil in a skillet over moderate heat until garlic softens. Add chicken broth and beans and simmer until most of the liquid is evaporated. Season with salt and pepper and serve with toasted pita.

Approx. 179 calories per serving
9g protein, 6g fat, 27g carbohydrates,
0 cholesterol, 702 mg sodium, 10g fiber

SAUTÉED PORTABELLOS WITH GARLIC AND PARSLEY

Ingredients: Makes 4 servings

2 tablespoons extra-virgin olive oil
12 oz. portabello mushrooms, cut into chunks
Salt and freshly ground pepper to taste
4 cloves fresh garlic, finely minced
1 tablespoon finely chopped parsley

In a skillet heat oil and sauté mushrooms over high heat for about 4 minutes. Add salt and pepper to taste. Sprinkle with garlic and parsley and serve hot.

Approx. 51 calories per serving
3g protein, 6g fat, 3g carbohydrates,
0 cholesterol, 3mg sodium, 0 fiber

GRILLED EGGPLANT

Ingredients: Makes 4 servings

1 tablespoon extra-virgin olive oil
2 tablespoons fresh oregano leaves
2 plum tomatoes, diced
1 1/2 lb. eggplant, cut lengthwise into 1/2-inch thick slices
Olive oil spray
2 large garlic cloves, finely minced
1 teaspoon chopped dried rosemary
1/2 teaspoon salt
1/4 teaspoon freshly ground black pepper
1/4 cup crumbled feta cheese
Lemon wedges
Oregano sprigs for garnish

Heat grill to medium-high heat. Heat oil in saucepan, add oregano leaves and remove pan from heat. Add tomato to oregano and allow to bath in hot oil until ready to serve. Spray both sides of eggplant with olive oil spray, sprinkle with garlic, rosemary and salt and pepper and place on medium hot grill. Cover grill and cook eggplant until tender and browned on both sides, turning once. Remove eggplant to platter and drizzle with oregano tomato oil, and top with feta cheese. Garnish with lemon wedges and oregano sprigs.

> *Approx. 85 calories per serving*
> *2g protein, 5g fat, 10g carbohydrates,*
> *3mg cholesterol, 210mg sodium, 4g fiber*

WRAPS AND SANDWICHES

ROASTED RED PEPPER SANDWICH (great in pita pockets)

Ingredients: Makes enough for 1 whole pita loaf (two 1/2 pockets)

2 large pieces of roasted red pepper (already prepared)
1 oz. hard Parmesano Reggiano cheese, sliced in thin pieces
1/2 cup alfalfa sprouts
4-6 Romaine lettuce leaves, broken
Salt and freshly ground black pepper to taste
1 whole wheat pita loaf, split in half and toasted
Garnish with a few black olives

Split pita loaf in half, open pocket of each side of loaf and lightly toast. Insert 1 piece of roasted pepper into each 1/2 pita pocket; add 1/2 of cheese to each pocket as well as sprouts and lettuce, salt and pepper to taste. Serve garnished with black olives.

Approx. 145 calories per 1/2 pocket
8g protein, 4g fat, 20g carbohydrates,
11mg cholesterol, 215mg sodium, 3g fiber

To make roasted red peppers (makes 4-6 servings)

4 large red bell peppers
1 clove garlic, peeled and sliced
4 tablespoons extra-virgin olive oil
Salt and freshly ground black pepper to taste

Clean peppers and pat dry. Place pepper on moderately hot grill, turning often until skin is charred and blistered. Charring of entire skin takes

(Continued)

about 15-20 minutes for this to happen. Remove from grill and place peppers aside to cool. Rub off blackened skins. Cut each pepper in half, remove stalk and seeds and cut into 1/2-inch strips. Place strips in a bowl, add garlic, oil, salt and pepper to taste. Store in a sealed jar in refrigerator.

> **Approx. 116 calories per serving**
> **1g protein, 9g fat, 7g carbohydrates,**
> **0 cholesterol, 2mg sodium, 2g fiber**

LAMB WRAP

Ingredients: Makes 4 wraps

1/3 cup medium-grain bulgur
1/2 cup diced tomatoes
1/2 cup finely chopped fresh parsley
1/4 cup finely chopped fresh mint leaves, no stems
2 scallions, thinly sliced
Juice from 1/2 lemon
2 tablespoons extra-virgin olive oil
Salt and freshly ground black pepper to taste
1/2 tablespoon extra-virgin olive oil
2 cloves garlic, minced
1/2 lb. lean ground lamb
Salt and freshly ground pepper to taste
4 oz. plain non-fat yogurt
1 tablespoon chopped fresh mint
3/4 cup diced cucumbers
1 cup fresh chopped spinach leaves
4 oz. crumbled fat-free feta cheese
4 (6-inch) pita loaves (do not split open)

Cover bulgur in a bowl with fresh cold water to a depth of roughly 1/2 -inch. Let stand until water is absorbed about 30 minutes. Fluff with a fork to separate grains. Grains should be plump and slightly moist, if too moist, spread grains on towel, fold towel and squeeze to remove excess water. Combine tomatoes, parsley, mint and scallions. Add bulgur to vegetables and oil, gently toss. Squeeze lemon juice over tabbouleh and refrigerate while making lamb. Heat olive oil, sauté garlic, lamb, and pepper and salt over medium-high heat until browned.

(Continued)

Stirring constantly to crumble, drain well and set aside. Combine yogurt, cucumbers and mint in small bowl, stir well and set aside. Stack pita rounds and wrap in wax paper, microwave on high for 45 seconds. In a bowl combine lamb mixture, spinach and feta. Spoon 1/2 cup tabbouleh mixture and 1/4 lamb mixture in the center of each pita round. Top with yogurt mixture and roll up pita. To secure, wrap bottom portion of pita roll-up with wax paper.

> *Approx. 462 calories per wrap*
> *21g protein, 20g fat, 43g carbohydrates,*
> *43mg cholesterol, 635mg sodium, 5g fiber*

VEGGIE WRAP

Ingredients: Makes 6 wraps

Olive oil cooking spray
2 medium tomatoes cut into 1/2-inch thick slices
2 small cucumbers, sliced lengthwise into 1/2-inch thick slices
2 small onion cut into 1/2-inch thick slices
1 green pepper cut into strips
2 medium zucchini, sliced lengthwise into 1/2-inch thick slices
Extra-virgin olive oil to drizzle
3/4 tablespoon dried oregano, crumbled
1/4 tablespoon dried rosemary, crumbled
3/4 teaspoon dried thyme
1/2 can (7 oz.) garbanzo beans, rinsed and drained
1/4 teaspoon cumin, optional
Salt and freshly ground black pepper to taste
Alfalfa sprouts, optional
6 whole wheat flat bread, (8-10-inch) warmed

Preheat oven to 425 degrees. Spray non stick pan with cooking spray. Place tomatoes, cucumbers, onions, peppers, and zucchini on pan, drizzle with olive oil. Sprinkle with herbs and roast for 15-20 minutes at 425 degrees. Add beans to vegetable mixture, cumin, salt and pepper to taste and cook additional 15-20 minutes until tender. Fill warmed flat bread with bean and veggie mix, top with alfalfa sprouts, roll-up and serve.

> *Approx. 170 calories per wrap*
> *8g protein, 1g fat, 36g carbohydrates,*
> *0 cholesterol, 325mg sodium, 6g fiber*

STUFFED WHOLE WHEAT KHUTZ (pita bread)

Ingredients: Makes 8 (1/2 pockets)

4 large (6-inch diameter) pita loaves
2 tablespoons stone ground mustard
1 teaspoon finely chopped fresh cilantro
2 cloves garlic, finely crushed
1/8 teaspoon ground cracked pepper
Sprinkle garlic salt to taste
1 1/2 teaspoons extra-virgin olive oil
1/4 teaspoon balsamic glaze
1/2 medium red onion, finely sliced
10 medium pitted black olives
1 1/2 cups shredded lettuce
1/2 cup chopped carrot
1/2 cup diced celery
1 large tomato, diced
4 oz. feta cheese, crumbled

Split 6-inch pita loaves crosswise in half, spread open pockets (to keep from sealing shut) and lightly toast. Lightly spread inside of toasted pockets with mustard. Set aside. Mix cilantro, garlic, pepper and salt with olive oil and glaze, stir together to blend well, set aside. Combine onion, olives, lettuce, carrots, celery, tomatoes, toss to mix and fill pockets with vegetable blend. Drizzle each stuffed loaf with glaze mixture, add crumbled feta. Serve.

> Approx. 152 calories per 1/2 loaf
> 6g protein, 7g fat, 18g carbohydrates,
> 12mg cholesterol, 353mg sodium, 3g fiber

SPICY HUMMUS IN TOASTED PITA LOAVES

Ingredients: Makes 6 (1/2 loaves) 6-inch round pita pockets

1 (15 oz.) can chickpeas, well rinsed and drained
Juice from 1 lemon
1/4 cup water
1 large garlic clove
2 tablespoons Tahini paste (Sesame seed paste)
Dash of salt
Pinch of red hot pepper flakes
3 (6-inch) round pita loaves- split in halves
8 slices tomatoes, 1/4-inch thick each
1/2 cucumber peeled, sliced thinly
Alfalfa sprouts

In a food process or blender add chickpeas, lemon juice and water, blend to desired consistency. Add garlic, Tahini paste, salt and hot pepper flakes, blend again. Cut pita loaves in half, toast lightly. Divide mixture into four portions and stuff loaves with mixture. Top each half loaf with tomato, cucumber and alfalfa sprouts.

> *Approx. 195 calories per stuffed 1/2 loaf pita pocket*
> *7g protein, 5g fat, 30g carbohydrates,*
> *0 cholesterol, 247 mg sodium, 0 fiber*

CHICKPEA PITA POCKETS

Ingredients: Makes filling for 8 half pockets

1 (15 oz.) can chickpeas, rinsed and drained
1 cup shredded fresh spinach
2/3 cup seedless red grapes, halved
1/2 cup finely chopped red bell pepper
1/3 cup thinly sliced celery
1/2 medium cucumber, diced
1/4 cup finely chopped onion
1/4 cup light mayonnaise
1 tablespoon balsamic syrup
1/2 tablespoon poppy seed
4 pita bread loaves slit in half crosswise

In a large bowl combine chickpeas, spinach, grapes, red pepper, celery, cucumber and onion. Whisk together mayonnaise, balsamic syrup and poppy seeds. Add poppy seed mixture to chickpea mixture, stir until well blended. Lightly toast pita halves and fill with chickpea filling. Serve

Approx. 178 calories per 1/2 loaf pita pocket
6g protein, 5g fat, 30g carbohydrates,
0 cholesterol, 413mg sodium, 4g fiber

SPICY MUSHROOM WRAP

Ingredients: Makes 2 wraps

Olive oil cooking spray
1 tablespoon extra-virgin olive oil
2 large portabello mushrooms, sliced
2 teaspoon minced fresh garlic
1/2 small white onion, thinly sliced
2 (10-inch) tortilla
2 teaspoons spicy brown mustard
1/2 lb. arugula, trimmed and steamed
10 cherry tomatoes, halved
1/4 cup shredded part-skim mozzarella cheese
1/2 hot cherry pepper, diced, optional

Preheat oven to 350 degrees. Spray baking dish with cooking spray. In a large skillet, heat olive oil, sauté mushrooms and garlic and onion for about 5 minutes, stirring constantly. Put mustard, arugula, tomato, and mozzarella and cooked mushroom mixture on each tortilla. Sprinkle hot peppers down center if desired; roll up and place seam-side down in oiled baking dish. Bake uncovered for 10 minutes or until cheese is melted. Serve.

Approx. 357 calories per serving
9g protein, 7g fat, 42g carbohydrates,
7mg cholesterol, 443mg sodium, 2g fiber

CHICKPEA AND FRESH SPINACH SANDWICH

Ingredients: Makes 4 servings

1 (15 oz.) can chickpeas, rinsed, drained and mashed to a paste
2 teaspoons extra-virgin olive oil
2 cloves fresh garlic, minced
1 clove fresh garlic, cut in half
1/2 medium white onion, diced
Salt to taste
Fresh ground pepper to taste
Red pepper flakes if desired
5-6 oz. fresh spinach leaves
8 slices whole wheat grain bread

Rinse and drain chickpeas thoroughly. Mash to a paste consistency, and set aside. In 1 teaspoon olive oil, sauté 2 cloves minced garlic and diced onion until golden brown. Add chickpeas paste, salt and pepper to taste, and red pepper flakes if desired. Drizzle paste with remaining teaspoon oil and set aside. Toast whole wheat bread slices and rub one side of each toast with fresh garlic halves. Divide paste mixture and spinach leaves into 4 portions and make into 4 sandwiches. Serve.

Approx. 216 calories per sandwich
15g protein, 6g fat, 38g carbohydrates,
0 cholesterol, 569 mg sodium, 14g fiber

SMOKED FISH AND ROASTED PEPPER SANDWICH

Ingredients: Makes 4 servings

2 tablespoons extra-virgin olive oil
8 slices whole wheat grain bread
1 clove fresh garlic, mashed to a paste
3 oz. smoked white fish
3 oz. smoked sturgeon
4 tablespoons Romaine lettuce
4 teaspoons diced roasted peppers
2 teaspoons light mayonnaise

Combine oil and garlic, reserving 1 teaspoon. Lightly brush both sides of bread with mixture and toast in oven at 350 degrees for 4 minutes or until golden brown. Set aside. Mix fish, lettuce and roasted peppers together, set aside. Blend mayo and 1 teaspoon oil together, add to fish mixture. Divide mixture into 4 servings and spread onto bread, making 4 sandwiches.

> *Approx. 232 calories per sandwich*
> *19g protein, 9g fat, 20g carbohydrates,*
> *24mg cholesterol, 618mg sodium, 4g fiber*

BREAD

Wheat flour is the most common variety of flour used for making bread, however other types such as barley flour, bran, buckwheat flour, cornmeal, rolled oats, oat flour, and soy flour to mention just a few are also suitable for bread making. All flours should be stored in airtight containers. All-purpose and white bread flour can be stored at 70 degrees F. for up to six months. Any flour, wheat or otherwise which contains the germ from the grain can easily turn rancid. These flours should be stored in the refrigerator or freezer and can be kept for up to three months.

MEDITERRANEAN CRUSTY-COUNTRY BREAD

Ingredients: Makes 1 loaf (1/2-inch thick slices)

To make Italian starter dough:
1/8 teaspoon active dry yeast
1/8 cup plus 1/2 cup lukewarm water
3/4 cup durum whole-wheat flour
1/2 cup unbleached white flour

Dissolve yeast in 1/8 cup warm water. Stir in remaining water. Add flour; mix with a wooden spoon for about 5 minutes until dough is sticky. Transfer dough to lightly oiled bowl, cover with plastic wrap and let rise at room temperature for about 24 hours. After 24 hours add to starter 1 teaspoon active yeast dissolved in 1 cup tepid water, 2 teaspoons salt and 2 cups of rye or whole wheat flour. Stir and mix thoroughly with hands. Cover bowl and return to a cool place for about 10 minutes. After 10 minutes, place to rise again in a warm place overnight. Next day add another 1 1/2 cups of tepid water and 1 cup of whole wheat flour and 1 cup of unbleached white flour. Begin kneading in a bowl, sprinkle flour on a pastry board and turn dough out. Knead for at least 10 minutes, adding flour until dough has an elastic consistency. Rinse bowl and dry and dust with flour. Place dough back into bowl and cover with plastic wrap. Set aside at room temperature for about 2-3 hours. After 2-3 hours turn dough out on lightly floured board-push down and kneed briefly. Form into a round ball or a long loaf and place on baking sheet, lightly sprinkle with cornmeal. Set aside in a warm place for 30 minutes.
Preheat oven to 450 degrees. Before baking slash loaf in 3-4 places (1/4 to 1/2-inch deep) with a sharp knife and immediately place in oven. Bake for 45 minutes until dark brown and crust is hard. Remove from oven and cool.

Approx. 80 calories per 1/2-inch slice
3g protein, 0 fat, 17g carbohydrates,
0 cholesterol, 147mg sodium, 0 fiber

FOCACCIA

A popular Italian bread found all over Italy. Usually round or rectangular in shape and about 1/2-1 inch thick. A variety of different toppings are used such as herbs, coarse salt or maybe a sprinkling of rosemary with hot pepper or perhaps olives or even an array of vegetables.

Ingredients: Makes 1 (11 1/2 x 17-inch Focaccia)

1 1/4 cup hot water
1 package rapid rising active dry yeast
1 tablespoon extra-virgin olive oil
3 tablespoons toasted wheat germ
Pinch salt
2 cups durum whole wheat flour plus extra for kneading
Olive oil for brushing surfaces

Preheat oven to 450 degrees. Pour water into a medium sized bowl and sprinkle with yeast. Stir with a wire whisk. Add wheat germ and olive oil and pinch of salt and whisk again. Add flour stir with a wooden spoon until dough forms a ball and leaves sides of bowl. Knead briefly add extra flour if needed until dough is no longer sticky but still soft, about 3 minutes. Turn dough out onto lightly floured surface; roll out into rectangle, 11x17-inch size. Lightly dust top with flour while rolling to prevent sticking. Ease dough into a lightly oiled 11x17-inch baking pan, stretch to fit and cover dough with sheet of lightly oiled waxed paper, oiled side down to allow to rise in a warm place for 25 minutes. After dough has risen, press down dough with your index finger to create little dimples over the surface. Add your favorite topping and bake in oven until lightly browned on the bottom, about 20-25 minutes. Remove and cool on rack. Slice into 12 large squares and serve.

> *Approx. 111 calories per square*
> *4g protein, 1g fat, 23g carbohydrates,*
> *0 cholesterol, 239mg sodium, 1g fiber*

EGYPTIAN KHUBZ (Pita bread)

The Arabs eat bread with every meal. They use it to scoop up sauces, dips, yogurt and liquids. Pita cut in half can be filled with shish kabobs, falafel or salads. They consider bread to be a divine gift from God.

Ingredients: Makes 12 loaves of pita

1 package dried yeast
1 1/2 cups warm water
1/4 teaspoon honey
1/2 tablespoon extra-virgin olive oil
Pinch of salt
4 cups durum whole wheat flour
Cornmeal to dust baking sheet

Dissolve yeast and honey in 1cup warm water and set aside for 5 minutes. Mix flour, salt and oil in a large bowl, add yeast mixture and remaining water and mix well. Knead for 10 minutes until dough is elastic; then place dough in a warm, oiled bowl, cover with a dry cloth and set in a warm place to double its volume (about 2-3 hours). Punch dough down and knead again for about 2 more minutes. Form dough into 12 smooth balls the size of oranges. Place balls on a dry cloth in a warm place and cover to rise for another 30 minutes. Preheat oven to 500 degrees and lightly flour a board with cornmeal and roll out balls into 1/4-inch thick circles. Bake loaves 5-8 minutes on a preheated baking sheet on center rack of oven. The loaves will puff up while baking but will collapse when cooled.

> *Approx. 218 calories per loaf*
> *7g protein, 3g fat, 41g carbohydrates,*
> *0 cholesterol, 497mg sodium, 10g fiber*

LAVOSH

Ingredients: Same as Pita Bread

Same recipe as for pita bread except leave pita bread in oven until it is golden brown and crisps, once cooled, break bread into pieces.
Same approx calories

SESAME BREAD (KERSA)

(A Moroccan type of round flat bread that is slightly crunchy on the outside and chewy on the inside.) Great for dipping in soup or with stews.

Ingredients: Makes 2 (16-inch round loaves) or 12 slices/ loaf

1 package of active dry yeast
1/4 cup plus 2 cups warm water
1 teaspoon granulated sugar or Splenda Granular
4 cups durum whole wheat Semolina flour
2 teaspoons salt
1/3 cup cornmeal and extra for dusting
1/2 tablespoon extra-virgin olive oil
2 teaspoon sesame seeds

Using a small bowl, combine yeast with 1/4 cup water, add sugar and let set until mixture starts to bubble. In a heavy duty mixer bowl with dough hook mix flour, 1/3 cup cornmeal and salt. Indent center of dough, pour in yeast mixture and olive oil. Knead dough adding remaining water as needed until dough takes on an elastic quality. Grease 2 baking sheets and dust with cornmeal. Separate dough to form 2 round balls and place each ball on a separate baking sheet. Press them into 8-inch circles. Sprinkle 1 teaspoon of sesame seeds over top of each loaf, gently pressing them into surface of dough. Cover dough with a clean cloth and set aside in a warm place for about 1 hour until they double their size. Preheat oven to 425 degrees. Prick the top of loaves with a fork and bake for 10 minutes. Lower heat to 375 degrees and bake loaves until top is crusty and golden brown, about 15-20 minutes.

> *Approx. 84 calories per slice*
> *3g protein, 1g fat, 16g carbohydrates,*
> *0 cholesterol, 90 mg sodium, 1g fiber*

DESSERTS

FRESH FRUITS AND NUTS PLATTER

A platter of seasonal fresh fruits such as bananas, Kiwi, figs, dates, strawberries, grapes, peaches, plums, pears, melons, apples, pomegranates, currants, mandarin oranges and various types of nuts could be served piled high on a platter alone or in mixed company. Fresh fruit simply often ends a Mediterranean meal. Sometimes these fruits are served in their dried form. Another great way to serve fresh fruit is as a fruit salad.

When using Splenda in a recipe, note that there are 2 types of Splenda. The Splenda in packets and Splenda Granulars. The Splenda in packet is somewhat sweeter tablespoon for tablespoon than the Granular type, however the Granular type is best for cooking. Splenda actually comes from sugar but has no calories. It measures equally tablespoon for tablespoon like sugar.

STRAWBERRY AND POACHED PEARS

Ingredients: Makes 4 servings

4 large ripe Anjou or Bartlett pears, peeled and cored
2 tablespoons fresh lemon juice
1 1/2 cups red wine (not cooking wine)
1 1/2 cups water
2 tablespoons Splenda Granulars
1 cinnamon stick
1 teaspoon orange rind, freshly grated
1/2 teaspoon lemon rind, freshly grated
1/4 teaspoon cloves, grounded
1 pint of fresh strawberries, cleaned and sliced
3 tablespoons Splenda (packets)
1 teaspoon Grand Marnier liqueur
Fresh mint leaves for garnish

Slice off bottom of pears to allow them to sit flat in a pan. Brush body of pears with lemon juice. In a saucepan combine wine, water, Splenda, cinnamon, orange rind, lemon rind and cloves in a sauce pan. Bring to a boil over medium heat, reduce heat and simmer for 5 minutes. Add pears, cover and poach for 20 minutes until tender. Let pears stand in liquid until cool. Refrigerate until ready to serve. When serving place pears on dessert plates and drizzle with a small amount of strawberry sauce. Garnish with mint leaf.

To make strawberry sauce:
Put strawberries in bowl and sprinkle with Splenda packets and Grand Marnier. Let stand at room temperature for 1 hour. Blend or process until pureed. Refrigerate sauce to chill.

> *Approx. 61 calories per serving*
> *2g protein, 0 fat, 16g carbohydrates,*
> *9g cholesterol, 1mg sodium,   6g fiber*

FIGS IN PLAIN YOGURT

Ingredients: Makes 4 servings

16 small figs
1 1/2 cups red wine
2 tablespoons honey
1/4 teaspoon ground cinnamon
2 cups plain low-fat yogurt
Splenda (packets) as desired
Finely chopped fresh mint for garnish

Slice open skins of figs on one side. Combine wine, honey, and cinnamon in a large saucepan and bring mixture to boil. Reduce to simmer, add figs and simmer for 10-15 minute. Remove from heat and allow figs to bath in liquid for 5-10 minutes. Remove skins from figs and mash figs. Combine mashed figs with yogurt and mix well, add Splenda if desired. Refrigerate until well chilled. Divide yogurt mixture into 4 dessert bowls. Sprinkle each with fresh mint.

Approx. 200 calories per serving
5g protein, 17g fat, 38g carbohydrates,
15mg cholesterol, 75mg sodium, 4g fiber

HONEY MOUSSE DELIGHT

Ingredients: Makes 6 servings

1/3 cup honey
2 teaspoons freshly grated orange rind
12 oz. part skim-milk ricotta cheese
2 1/2 cups halved fresh strawberries
2 1/2 cups blackberries
1/4 cup fresh orange juice
3 tablespoons Splenda (packets)
2 tablespoons finely chopped walnuts

Mix honey, rind and ricotta cheese in a medium bowl; cover and refrigerate to chill. Combine berries, juice, splenda, gently toss and let stand for 5 minutes before covering and re-chilling. When well chilled, spoon 1/3 berry mixture (divided equally) into six serving bowls and top each with about 1/4 cup of ricotta mixture. Divide remaining fruit mixture evenly among each serving on top of cheese. Sprinkle each serving with nuts and serve.

> *Approx. 188 calories per serving*
> *7g protein, 5g fat, 31g carbohydrates,*
> *29mg cholesterol, 71mg sodium, 5g fiber*

SPICE CAKE

Ingredients: Makes 1 (3x5-inch) loaf

1/2 teaspoon anise seed
3/4 cups water
1/2 cup honey
1/2 cup Splenda Granulars
1/2 teaspoon baking soda
3 cups unbleached white flour
1/8 teaspoon cinnamon
1/4 teaspoon fresh grated nutmeg
1/8 cup mixed orange and lemon peels, chopped
Pinch of salt
Olive Oil Spray

Preheat oven to 350 degrees. In a medium sauce pan bring anise seed, covered with water to a boil, add honey and Splenda, stir until both are dissolved. Remove mixture from heat and add baking soda. Sift flour, spices and salt into a large bowl. Add orange and lemon peels. Strain liquid from anise seeds and mix into dry ingredients, stirring all the time. Beat until mixture is smooth. Pour mixture into 3x5-inch sprayed and floured baking pan and bake for 1 hour, or until cake just begins to shrink from sides of pan. Remove from oven and let cool slightly. Serve warm or cool.

Approx. 341 calories per 1-inch slice
49g protein, 0 fat, 59g carbohydrates,
0 cholesterol, 126mg sodium, 0 fiber

BAKLAVA

Ingredients: Makes 24 pieces

1 1/2 cups Splenda Granulars
3/4 cup water
2 tablespoons rose water
3 3/4 cups chopped, unsalted mixed nuts (such as walnuts, almonds, hazelnuts)
1/4 cup Splenda Granulars
1 teaspoon ground cinnamon
1 1/4 stick butter, melted
1-16 oz. package frozen Filo pastry, thawed

To make syrup: Boil 1 1/2 cups splenda with 3/4 cup water for about 2 minutes, take care not to let it burn or boil over. Before removing it from heat stir in 2 tablespoons rose water. Let cool and refrigerate until ready for use.

For Baklava: Preheat oven to 325 degrees. Combine in a small bowl nuts, splenda and cinnamon. Lightly brush a 12x17-inch baking pan with melted butter. Layer sheets of filo dough; buttering each as it's layered over other. Spread top sheet evenly with 1/3 nut mixture. Cover nut mixture with three more sheets of filo dough, brush each sheet with butter. Repeat these layers 2 more times, covering last nut layer with remaining filo dough. With a sharp knife carefully score the top layers of pastry into 24 squares or diamond shapes. Bake in 325 degree oven for 30 minutes. Increase oven temperature to 350 degrees and continue baking until pastry is golden brown and puffed, about 10 minutes. Remove pastry from oven; pour cold syrup over hot pastry. Set aside to room temperature before serving.

Approx. 191 calories per piece
5g protein, 18g fat, 4g carbohydrates,
17mg cholesterol, 164mg sodium, 2g fiber

PEACH MARSALA COMPOTE

Ingredients: Makes 6 servings

1? fresh peaches
6 cups water
3/4 cup Splenda Granulars
1/2 cup Marsala wine
1/2 teaspoon ground cinnamon
1/2 teaspoon vanilla extract
1/2 teaspoon freshly grated nutmeg
Olive Oil Spray

Preheat oven to 350 degrees. Lightly spray a 2 quart baking dish with cooking spray. Blanch the peaches in boiling water for 20 seconds. Remove peaches from pot and while holding under running cold water, remove the skins. Pit and slice peaches. Add peaches, Splenda, wine, cinnamon, extract and nutmeg to a baking dish and bake for 45 minutes to 1 hour. Serve warm or at room temperature.

> *Approx. 164 calories per serving*
> *2g protein,   0 fat, 40g carbohydrates,*
> *0 cholesterol, 1mg sodium, 4g fiber*

SWEET PLUM COMPOTE

Ingredients: Makes 6 servings

3 lbs. ripe plums, halved and pitted
1/4 cup Splenda Granulars
1 cup water
1 tablespoon crème de cassis liqueur
Olive Oil Spray

Preheat oven to 350 degrees. Lightly spray a baking dish with cooking spray. Add plums to baking dish. Combine Splenda and water in a saucepan and bring to a boil, cook for about 5 minutes, stirring constantly, or until liquid becomes syrupy. Pour syrup over plums and drizzle with crème de cassis. Bake mixture for 45 minutes to 1 hour. Serve warm or cool.

> *Approx. 158 calories per serving*
> *2g protein, 2g fat, 37g carbohydrates,*
> *0 cholesterol, 0 sodium, 2g fiber*

YOGURT NUT CAKE

Ingredients: Makes 1 (9x13-inch) cake or 13 (1-inch thick) slices

1 cup Splenda Granulars
1 lb. melted butter, cooled
4 eggs, beaten
1 1/2 cups plain yogurt
1/2 teaspoon baking soda
1/2 cup milk
3 cups unbleached flour, sifted
1 teaspoon baking powder
1/4 pound walnuts, chopped (1cup)
2 cups Splenda Granulars for syrup
1 cup water

To make syrup: Stir sugar and water together in a heavy saucepan over medium heat until sugar dissolves. Bring syrup to a boil, stirring often. Remove from heat and cool in refrigerator.

For cake: Preheat oven to 350 degrees. Add sugar slowly to melted butter and mix thoroughly. Add beaten egg, mixing well. Stir in yogurt. Combine baking soda, milk and add to yogurt mixture. Combine sifted flour and baking powder and blend into yogurt mixture, 1 cup at a time. Blend vigorously until thoroughly blended. Pour batter into floured pan and bake at 350 degrees for 1 hour or until cake is golden brown on top. While cake is still hot cut into 1-inch thick slices and sprinkle nuts over the top. Spoon cool syrup over each piece and serve.

> *Approx. 442 calories per slice with syrup*
> *8g protein, 34g fat, 25g carbohydrates,*
> *146mg cholesterol, 333mg sodium, 0 fiber*

SWEET MANGO MOUSSE

Ingredients: Makes 6 servings

1 1/4 cups water
1 cup couscous
4 tablespoons Splenda (packets)
3/4 cup fresh juice oranges
2 tablespoons orange-flavored liqueur
1 large ripe mango
1 cup heavy whipping cream, well chilled
1 1/4 teaspoons vanilla extract
1 (8 oz.) container vanilla yogurt
Orange zest, finely minced for garnish

Bring water to a boil over medium-high heat. Add couscous slowly, stirring once and remove from heat. Cover and set aside for 12-15 minutes until couscous is tender. Add 2 tablespoons of Splenda, mix well into couscous. Cover and set aside. In a small saucepan over medium, heat orange juice, stirring constantly until reduced to the consistency of honey (about 4-5 minutes). Stir in liqueur. Set aside. Peel the mango; cut half of flesh into thin wedges and the other half coarsely dice and set aside. Pour cream into a chilled bowl and whip until it peaks. Fold in vanilla and remaining Splenda. Divide in half. Save half for serving. In a clean bowl, combine remaining half of whipped cream, yogurt and diced mango refrigerate until well chilled. Before serving, combine mango mixture with couscous. Divide into 6 equal portions. Top each portion with a good dollop of the remaining whipped cream and mango wedges. Drizzle with liqueur sauce and sprinkle with minced orange zest.

> Approx. 310 calories per serving
> 7g protein, 15g fat, 38g carbohydrates,
> 51mg cholesterol, 43mg sodium, 2g fiber

FRESH FRUIT KABOBS AND CINNAMON HONEY DIP

Ingredients: Makes 2 servings (1 fruited skewer and 1 cup of dip per person)

Assorted bite sized chunks of your favorite fresh fruits- such as apples, peaches, pears, pineapple, cantaloupe, kiwi (enough mixed chunks for 2 (8-inch) wooden skewers)
2 cups of plain yogurt
2 tablespoons of honey or Splenda Granulars
Pinch of ground white pepper
6 teaspoons of ground cinnamon or to taste

Prepare fruits on skewers. Set aside. Combine yogurt, honey, white pepper mix well. Divide mixture into two individual serving bowls, sprinkle cinnamon on top of each serving and gently swirl in, cover and refrigerate to chill before serving.

FRESH FRUIT IN YOGURT WITH RUM

(your favorite liqueur can be substituted for rum if desired)

Ingredients: Makes 2 servings

**1/4 cup each of blueberries and sliced strawberries or sliced grapes, kiwi or raspberries
2 cups plain yogurt
Dark Rum to taste
Splenda (packets) to taste if desired**

Cut up enough desired fresh fruit for 2 servings; add 2 cups plain yogurt and mix well. Divide mixture into two individual glass dessert cups and generously splash each serving with dark rum. Add sweetener if desired, chill before serving.

*Approx. 110 calories per serving
13g protein, 0 fat, 15g carbohydrates,
0 cholesterol, 80mg sodium, 0 fiber*

STUFFED DATES

Ingredients: Makes 16

16 pitted dates
16 whole almonds
6 tablespoons almond paste

Slice dates open on one side. Pull back skin from the meat of the date and stuff each date with one almond and 1 teaspoon almond paste. Serve

SWEET ITALIAN RICE PUDDING

Ingredients: Makes 6 servings

24 oz. evaporated skim milk
1/4 cup long grain rice
3 tablespoons Splenda Granulars
1 teaspoon vanilla extract
Ground cinnamon

Combine 12 oz. milk and rice in a double boiler over simmering water. Cook stirring frequently for about 20 minutes. Add remaining milk and Splenda, mix well. Simmer stirring often until pudding consistency, about 45 minutes. Add 1 teaspoon vanilla extract, blend into pudding while simmering for an additional few minutes. Remove from heat and sprinkle generously with cinnamon. Cool to room temperature, cover and refrigerate before serving.

> *Approx. 117 calories per serving*
> *8g protein, 0 fat, 15g carbohydrates,*
> *4mg cholesterol, 24mg sodium, 0 fiber*

CRÈME DE BANANA BAKED APPLES

Ingredients: Makes 4-6 servings

4 medium sweet apples, peeled, cored and halved
6 oz. unsweetened apple juice
2 teaspoons ground cinnamon
3 tablespoons pure honey
1 teaspoon vanilla extract
4 tablespoons Crème de Banana liqueur
1 cup plain fat free yogurt
Splenda (packets) to taste

Preheat oven to 350 degrees. Place apples cored side up in a snugly fitting shallow baking dish. Add apple juice to just barely cover bottom halves of apples. Sprinkle with 1 teaspoon cinnamon, cover and bake for 30-40 minutes, or until apples are almost tender. Remove from oven and pour off any additional liquid leaving just enough to cover bottom of dish. Drizzle tops of apples with honey, extract, liqueur and remaining teaspoon of cinnamon. Bake for an additional 10 minutes. Remove from oven and divide equally onto 4 dessert plates. Blend yogurt and Splenda together and serve to the side of apples.

Approx. 128 calories per serving
2g protein, 0 fat, 28g carbohydrates,
1mg cholesterol, 31mg sodium, 6g fiber

CANTALOUPE SORBET

Ingredients: Makes 4-6 servings (Other sorbets can be made using this recipes. The best fruits to use are very ripe fruits like mangoes, pears or berries)

1 1/2 cups of water
1/2 cup Splenda (packets)
2 ripe cantaloupes, peeled, halved, seeded and chunked
1/4 cup fresh lemon juice
egg white from 1 large egg
Mint sprigs for garnish

Combine water and Splenda, bring to a boil over medium heat. Reduce heat and simmer for 5 minutes, allow too cool. In a food processor or blender add cantaloupe and its juices, lemon juice, and cooled syrup. Puree until smooth. Pour mixture into bowl and freeze until almost frozen. Remove from freezer and beat with an electric beater until mixture is again smooth. Beat egg white until stiff and fold into frozen fruit mixture. Cover container and freeze again until firm (about 2-3 hours). When ready to serve, scoop into dessert cups and garnish with mint sprig if desired.

Approx. 98 calories per serving
2g protein, 0 fat, 24g carbohydrates,
0 cholesterol, 24mg sodium, 2g fiber

HONEYDEW SORBET

Ingredients: Same as cantaloupe sorbet but use honeydew instead. Follow same directions.

STRAWBERRIES AND BALSAMIC SYRUP

Ingredients: Makes 4 servings

2 1/2 cups strawberries, hulled and halved
4 tablespoons crème de banana liqueur
Splenda packets
Balsamic syrup

Combine strawberries and crème de banana in a large bowl, toss well, cover and refrigerate 20-30 minutes. When ready to serve, remove strawberries with a slotted spoon and place as a single layer on a dessert platter, dust generously with Splenda and drizzle with balsamic syrup.

> *Approx. 65 calories per serving*
> *1g protein, 0 fat, 11g carbohydrates,*
> *0 cholesterol, 2mg sodium, 2g fiber*

DRUNKEN PEACHES

Ingredients: Makes 4 servings

4 peaches
1 1/2 cups red wine
1 1/3 cups water
3 strips lemon peel (yellow only)
3 tablespoons honey
1 cinnamon stick
Sprinkle with Splenda to taste (optional)
Fat-free whipped cream (optional)

Peel skin from peaches. In a sauce pan add wine, water, lemon peel, honey and cinnamon stick and bring to boil. Add peaches to sauce, submerge under liquid as much as possible and gently poach for 5-10 minutes until just tender. Remove peaches from sauce pan and place in a bowl, set aside. Boil liquid in the sauce pan, stirring constantly until it becomes thick and syrupy. Remove cinnamon stick and lemon peel before liquid becomes dark. Pour syrup, when cool, over peaches and serve. Garnish with Splenda and whipped cream if desired.

> *Approx. 156 calories per serving*
> *1g protein, 0 fat, 24g carbohydrates,*
> *0 cholesterol, 0 sodium, 2g fiber*

DRUNKEN APRICOTS

Ingredients: Makes 4 servings

Same recipe as above for Drunken peaches, except use 8 medium sized apricots.

> **Approx. 148 calories per serving**
> **0 protein, 0 fat, 21g carbohydrates,**
> **0 cholesterol, 0 sodium, 1g fiber**

SPICED APPLES

Ingredients: Makes 4-6 servings

1/8 cup Splenda
1/8 teaspoon cinnamon
6 small apples
1 1/2 teaspoons light corn syrup
1 1/2 cups dry white wine
1/2 + 1/4 cup apple cider
Dash nutmeg
1/2 teaspoon finely shredded orange peel

Preheat oven to 400 degrees. Combine Splenda and cinnamon. Roll apples in corn syrup, then in cinnamon/Splenda mixture. Place apples in a baking dish, bake at 400 degrees for 15 minutes. Combine wine, cider, nutmeg and orange peel, heat on low-heat. Pour over baked apples and serve.

> **Approx. 179 calories per serving**
> **0 protein, 0 fat, 3g carbohydrates,**
> **0 cholesterol, 4mg sodium, 4g fiber**

STRAWBERRIES AMARETTO

Ingredients: Makes 8 servings

1 1/2 quart strawberries, halved except for 8 strawberries
2 cups plain low-fat yogurt
1 teaspoon vanilla extract
1/4 cup amaretto liqueur
Fat-free whipped cream (if desired)

Set aside 8 strawberries for garnish. Hull remaining ones and cut into halves. Place strawberry halves in dessert glasses. In a bowl, combine yogurt, extract and amaretto, blend well. Pour amaretto mixture over strawberries and garnish with reserved berries. Add whipped cream, if desired.

> *Approx. 85 calories per serving*
> *4g protein, 2g fat, 12g carbohydrates,*
> *3mg cholesterol, 46mg sodium, 2g fiber*

LEMON SHERBET

Ingredients: Makes 4-6 servings (make orange sherbet by using oranges instead of lemons)

3 large lemons, squeeze juice to get 2/3 cup fresh lemon juice
Peel from 3 lemons (yellow part only)
1/2 cup honey
2 1/2 cups water
Egg white from 1 egg

Remove peel from lemons, set aside. Squeeze all 3 lemons to get 2/3 cup of fresh lemon juice, set aside. In a sauce pan add zest, honey and water. Bring to a rapid boil for 5 minutes. Allow to cool to room temperature. Strain lemon juice through a sieve. When mixture has cooled, add strained lemon juice, pour into freezer container and freeze until mushy. When mushy, stir ice crystals from edges of container. Do this every hour for 4 hours. Remove from freezer and whisk until smooth. Beat egg white to stiffen and fold into whisked lemon mixture. Cover and return to freezer for another 2-3 hours, until it has the consistency of packed snow. Serve immediately.

> *Approx. 88 calories per serving*
> *0 protein, 0 fat, 23g carbohydrates,*
> *0 cholesterol, 9mg sodium, 0 fiber*

APPETIZERS, DIPS and SNACK FOODS

STUFFED GRAPE LEAVES (Dolmas)

Ingredients: Makes 20 servings

3 tablespoons extra-virgin olive oil
1 cup red onion, chopped
1/2 cup chopped scallions
1 cup basmati rice
4 garlic cloves, minced
1 teaspoon ground cumin
1/2 teaspoon freshly ground pepper
1 can (15 oz.) vegetable broth plus enough water to make 2 cups of liquid
1/4 cup chopped fennel
1/4 cup chopped dill
1/4 cup finely chopped parsley
2 tablespoons dried mint
1 (16 oz.) jar grape leaves
2 cups water

For sauce:
2 cups plain non-fat yogurt
4 scallions, minced
1 clove garlic, minced
1 teaspoon salt

In a skillet over medium heat add 1 tablespoon oil, onions and scallions. Cook until soft and transparent. Add rice, cook until grains are slightly browned, stirring constantly. Add garlic, cumin, pepper, and vegetable broth plus water. Reduce heat to simmer, cover and cook until rice is tender and all liquid is absorbed. Allow rice to cool, stir in fennel, dill,

(Continued)

parsley and mint. Set aside. Drain grape leaves and cover with water, bring to a rolling boil. Blanch leaves for 1-2 minutes, drain and allow too cool. With leaf shiny side down, fill 20 leaves with mixture and roll leaves starting at the stem and folding in sides as you roll until they neatly packaged. Repeat until all 20 leaves are filled. Line a heavy bottomed pan with 10 of the unfilled grape leaves. Pack the rolled leaves in tightly side by side with seam side down. Top rolled leaves with lemon slices and cover lemon slices with remaining unfilled grape leaves. Mix together water and remaining olive oil and pour over grape leaf rolls. Place an object like a heavy plate on top of rolls to help hold them below the water level during cooking. Simmer for about 1 hour, checking to make sure they haven't boiled dry. Remove pan from stove and allow too cool. Remove rolls from pan and chill. Serve chilled or at room temperature, garnished with lemon wedges or yogurt sauce.

For yogurt sauce:
Mix together, 2 cups plain yogurt, scallions, garlic and salt to taste. Chill until ready to serve.

> *Approx. 51 calories per serving*
> *2g protein, 2g fat, 6g carbohydrates,*
> *0 cholesterol, 115mg sodium, 0 fiber*

MARINATED OLIVES

3 oz. Manzanilla olives
3 oz. Kalamata olives
3 cloves crushed garlic
1 large bay leaf
1/2 teaspoon oregano
1/4 teaspoon rosemary
1/2 teaspoon ground cumin
1/2 teaspoon fennel seed
1/2 teaspoon thyme
4 tablespoons white vinegar

If olives are soaking in brim, drain brim from olives and rinse olives under cold water. Set olives aside. In a 7 oz. jar, place all other ingredients, add olives and water to top of jar and cap. Marinate at room temperature for 2 days.

Approx. 60 calories
6-8 medium olives

TOMATO AND GARLIC TOPPING FOR BRUSCHETTE

Ingredients: Makes enough for 8 Brochette slices

1 teaspoon extra-virgin olive oil
1 1/4 cups chopped plum tomatoes
1 1/2 teaspoons minced garlic
1 teaspoon balsamic vinegar
1/2 teaspoon dried basil
1/4 teaspoon Splenda
1/4 teaspoon ground pepper
8 (1/2 inch thick) slices of Baguette
     or French bread or crusty whole wheat

Place slices on ungreased baking sheet, brush each slice with olive oil and bake at 500 degrees for 3-4 minutes until lightly browned. Combine tomatoes, garlic, vinegar, basil, sugar and pepper in a small bowl. Mix well and spoon mixture over bread slices.

> *Approx. 72 calories per slice*
> *2g protein, 1g fat, 13g carbohydrates,*
> *1mg cholesterol, 12mg sodium, 0 fiber*

TOMATO AND FRESH PARMESAN CHEESE BRUSCHETTE TOPPING

Ingredients: Makes 8 slices

8 (1/2 inch thick) slices French bread or crusty whole wheat
   (scantly brushed with olive oil on both sides)
2 cloves garlic, finely minced
1 teaspoon extra-virgin olive oil
1 small onion, diced
1 medium tomato, diced
Pinch dried oregano, crumbled
Pinch fresh black pepper
2 tablespoons freshly grated Parmesan cheese

Preheat oven to 500 degrees. Scantly brush slices of bread on both sides with oil and toast. Remove from oven and evenly distribute garlic on one side of bread. Rub garlic into bread with handle of knife and set aside, keep warm. Heat teaspoon of oil in skillet, add onions and lightly sauté until golden brown. Remove from heat. Preheat broiler. Combine onion, tomatoes, oregano and pepper, spread evenly over garlic bread and sprinkle with cheese. Place bread with cheese under broiler for 1 minute until lightly browned. Serve immediately.

> *Approx. 68 calories per slice*
> *2g protein, 1g fat, 12g carbohydrates,*
> *1 mg cholesterol, 1mg sodium, 0 fiber*

ROASTED GARLIC

Ingredients: Makes 1 jumbo garlic (great for serving with bread or with vegetables)

1 jumbo garlic
Olive oil as needed

Preheat oven to 400 degrees. Cut off the point of jumbo garlic and place cut side up in a baking dish. Drizzle garlic with olive oil and bake in heated oven for 25 minutes or more until garlic is soft. Serve to mash as a spread on bread or eat as is. Great with cooked vegetables or fish.

QUICK GARLIC BRUSCHETTE

Ingredients:

1 loaf crusty country bread (page 223)
Cloves of garlic, peeled, and halved
Extra-virgin olive oil
Salt to taste
Milled ground cracked pepper

Slice desired amount of bread and toast slices. Rub toasted pieces and rub toasted slices with garlic cloves until cloves almost disappear. Drizzle garlicky toast with olive oil, sprinkle with salt and pepper. Serve.

ITALIAN CROSTINI (Great toppings: smoked mozzarella, chopped fresh tomatoes, chopped black olives, roasted red peppers, roasted garlic or chopped arugula)

Ingredients:

1 baguette, sliced in 1/3-inch thick rounds
2 large cloves garlic, peeled and halved
Extra- virgin olive oil
Minced dried or fresh basil, chervil, parsley or chives
Sea salt to taste
Milled ground cracked pepper

Preheat oven to 375 degrees. Rub baguette slices on one side generously with garlic halves. Brush slices lightly on both sides with olive oil. Add desired herb or combination of herbs, salt and pepper. Place slices on baking sheet and bake until golden on edges, about 3-5 minutes. Add your favorite topping to each slice if desired or serve as is.

CHILLED AVOCADO DIP

Ingredients: Makes 1 cup

4 tablespoons fresh lemon juice
3 tablespoons sesame seed paste (Tahini)
2 medium avocados, peeled and cut into pieces
1/4 cup finely chopped parsley
3 tablespoons extra-virgin olive oil
2 medium cloves garlic, crushed
Salt and pepper to taste
2 pinches cayenne
Sprinkling of paprika

Blend lemon juice and sesame seed paste, set aside. Add avocados, parsley, olive oil, garlic and cayenne. Transfer to serving bowl and add salt and pepper to taste. Refrigerate to chill. When ready to serve, sprinkle with paprika.

> *Approx. 1312 calories per 1 cup*
> *21g protein, 132g fat, 32g carbohydrates,*
> *0 cholesterol, 54mg sodium, 16g fiber*

HUMMUS DIP (chickpeas)

(A great dip for fresh vegetables and pita bread)

Ingredients: Makes 4 servings

1 can (19 oz.) chickpeas, drained, reserve 1/4 cup of liquid
1/2 cup sesame seed paste
6 tablespoons lemon juice
Salt and pepper to taste
3 tablespoons extra-virgin olive oil
1 tablespoon finely chopped fresh mint

Blend chickpeas with 1/4 cup liquid and sesame seed paste, lemon juice and salt into a smooth paste with the consistency of butter. If too thick, add water if necessary. Place on serving plate, drizzle with olive oil and garnish with mint.

> *Approx. 392 calories per serving*
> *13g protein, 31g fat, 24g carbohydrates,*
> *0 cholesterol, 130mg sodium, 0 fiber*

GREEK BEAN DIP

Ingredients: Makes 3 3/4 cups

2 (15 oz. each) cans great northern beans, rinsed and drained
1 (8 oz.) package cream cheese
4 oz. feta cheese
3 cloves minced garlic
2 tablespoons lemon juice
1 tablespoon chopped fresh oregano
1/2 teaspoon ground pepper
1/4 teaspoon salt
1/2 cup seeded tomato, finely chopped
1/4 cup sliced ripe olives

Process (food processor) beans, cream cheese, feta cheese, garlic, lemon juice, oregano, pepper and salt until smooth. Transfer mixture to a 1 1/2 quart baking dish, cover and bake at 350 degrees for 25 minutes or until heated through. Remove from heat and sprinkle tomato and olives over dip and serve.

> *Approx. 19 calories per tablespoon serving*
> *1 protein, 0 fat, 2g carbohydrates,*
> *1mg cholesterol, 86mg sodium, 0 fiber*

GREEK FETA AND WALNUT DIP

Great with toasted pita triangles or fresh fruit

Ingredients. Makes 2 cups

1/2 lb. feta cheese
2 tablespoons extra-virgin olive oil
2/3 cup milk
1 cup walnuts
Pinch cayenne
2 tablespoons minced parsley

Drain feta cheese, combine all ingredients in a food processor and process until smooth. Let mixture stand for 1 hour before serving.

SKORDALIA

Goes well with vegetables such as pea pods, zucchini, and cucumbers as a dip

Ingredients: Makes 2 1/2 cups

3 slices bread, crust removed
1 cup blanched almonds, finely chopped
6 cloves garlic, chopped fine
Salt to taste
3 tablespoons fresh lemon juice
3/4 cup extra-virgin olive oil

In a food processor, using metal blade chop bread into pieces. Add ground almonds, garlic and salt and continuing processing to form a paste. Add lemon juice and mix well. Add olive oil a few drops at a time, as you are processing until mixture becomes thick and creamy. Continue adding oil until mixture is light and fluffy. Transfer to serving bowl and serve.

HERB CUCUMBER YOGURT DIP

Great for dipping wedges of toasted pita or fresh raw vegetables

Ingredients: Makes 2 cups; 6 8 servings

1 English cucumber
2 cups plain yogurt
2 teaspoons white wine vinegar
2 cloves garlic, chopped
2 tablespoons extra-virgin olive oil
2 teaspoons dill
2 teaspoons dried mint
Salt and fresh ground pepper to taste
2 tablespoons fresh mint, chopped

Peel and slice cucumbers (if very seedy, remove seeds). Place in bowl and sprinkle with a little salt, let sit for about 15 minutes to draw out water. In a separate bowl, mash garlic into a paste, add pinch of salt, vinegar and oil, stir. Add yogurt, dill and dried mint, mix well. Rinse salt from cucumber slices and pat dry, removing any excess water. Combine cucumbers with yogurt mixture; add salt and fresh ground pepper to taste. Garnish with fresh chopped mint and serve.

Approx. 79 calories per serving
3g protein, 5g fat, 4g carbohydrates,
9mg cholesterol, 41mg sodium, 0 fiber

ROASTED PEPPER DIP

Serve with pita wedges or dipping or fresh raw vegetables

Ingredients: Makes 1 1/2 cups; about 6-8 servings

4 large red bell peppers
2 cloves garlic, peeled and minced
1 tablespoon red vinegar
3 tablespoons extra-virgin olive oil
Salt and fresh ground pepper to taste

Clean peppers and pat dry. Place pepper on moderately hot grill, turning often until skin is charred and blistered. Charring of entire skin takes about 15-20 minutes for this to happen. Remove from grill and place peppers aside to cool. Rub off blackened skins. Cut each pepper in half, remove stalk and seeds and cut into 1/2-inch strips. In a food processor add vinegar and pulse adding oil slowly until peppers are smooth. Transfer pepper mixture from processor to a bowl. Mash garlic and stir into pepper dip, add salt and pepper to taste.

> *Approx. 60 calories per serving*
> *0 protein, 5g fat, 5g carbohydrates,*
> *0 cholesterol, 2mg sodium, 2g fiber*

TOASTED TAHINI DIP

Serve with warmed pita wedges

Ingredients:

1/3 cup Tahini
3 tablespoons fresh lemon juice
1/4 teaspoon lemon zest
1 cup plain yogurt
1 clove garlic, pressed
1 tablespoon finely chopped scallions (green part only)
Pinch of salt
Pinch of cayenne
2 tablespoons toasted sesame seeds

Toast sesame seeds in a heavy skillet on high, stirring constantly so they do not burn. When seeds pop, remove from heat and spread out to cool. When cooled, add all ingredients together and mix well. Cover and chill. Serve with warmed pita wedges.

HUMMUS WITH TAHINI DIP

Ingredients: Makes about 2 cups

4 cups of canned chickpeas, rinsed and drained
3 tablespoons of Tahini
3 tablespoons of freshly squeezed lemon juice
4 cloves of garlic, crushed to a paste
Salt to taste
1 tablespoon fresh cilantro, chopped
4 tablespoons extra-virgin olive oil

Puree the peas in a food processor or blender. Blend together the Tahini, lemon juice, garlic and salt. Combine this to the chickpeas and blend until it is a smooth paste. Serve garnished with cilantro and drizzled with olive oil.

SPICES, SAUCES and DRESSINGS

HARISSA (RED PEPPER SPICE)

The Tunisian Kitchens are noted for spicy hotness (Harissa). This hot pepper sauce adds piquancy to all types of stews as well as couscous. If you are brave enough, it is even eaten on its own as a spread on bread. Commercial Harissa is imported from North Africa and is available in tubes found in most gourmet stores where couscous is sold.

Ingredients: Makes about 2/3 cup

1/2 cup ground fresh cayenne
5 cloves fresh garlic, peeled, crushed
2 tablespoons caraway seeds, finely ground
1 tablespoon water
1/4 cup cumin
1 teaspoon coriander seed
2 tablespoons salt
1/2 cup extra-virgin olive oil

Mix all spices together in a mortar. Add crushed garlic and salt to spice mixture and mash together to form a paste. Add water and 1/4 cup of olive oil in a jar and paste, mix well. Spoon remaining olive oil over the top, tightly cover and refrigerate. It keeps for months.

Approx. 129 calories per 1 tablespoon
0g protein, 11g fat, 4g carbohydrates,
0 cholesterol, 640mg sodium, 1g fiber)

THICK POMEGRANATE MOLASSES

Ingredients: Makes 1 cup

3 cups fresh pomegranate juice

In a 1 1/2 quart saucepan bring 3 cups of juice to a boil over medium heat. Reduce heat and simmer, uncovered, stirring occasionally and skimming the froth until juice is reduced to 1 cup. Cool, bottle and store in refrigerator.

> **Approx. 255 calories per 1 cup molasses**
> **3g protein, 0 fat, 63g carbohydrates, 0 cholesterol, 0 sodium, 0g fiber**

YOGURT DRESSING

Plain yogurt flavored with crushed garlic or spearmint to taste

SPICE RUB

Ingredients: Makes 1/--eat combination seasoning for fish)

2 tablespoons curry powder
1 tablespoon cumin powder
1 teaspoon sugar
1/2 teaspoon salt
1/2 teaspoon paprika
1/4 teaspoon cardamom

Combine together and dredge fish before cooking

MIXED SPICES

Ingredients: Makes about 2 tablespoons

2 teaspoons ground allspice
1 teaspoon ground cinnamon
1 teaspoon ground cloves
1 teaspoon ground coriander
1 teaspoon ground cumin
1/4 teaspoon freshly ground black pepper

Combine ingredients and store in a small jar with a tight lid in a cool dry place away from light.

BASIL PESTO SAUCE

This highly flavored sauce goes a long way. One spoonful of pesto is all that is needed to flavor minestrone, vegetables, grilled chicken, fish or pasta.

Ingredients: Makes 1 cup of sauce (enough for 6 servings of pasta)

1/3 cup pine nuts, toasted
2 1/2 cups fresh basil leaves
1 teaspoon lemon juice
1/4 teaspoon salt
4 cloves garlic
3/4 cup extra-virgin olive oil
3/4 cup grated Parmesan cheese or aged pecorino
Freshly ground black pepper to taste

In a small skillet toast pine nuts over medium heat for 1-2 minutes. Remove from heat, set aside. Cut basil leaves into strips. Combine lemon juice, salt and garlic in a mortar and mash into a paste. Add pine nuts and continue to mix until nuts are ground. Add basil strips a few at a time gradually grounding them into nut mixture. Add a splash of olive oil and mix until paste becomes loose. Add grated parmesan cheese, pepper and remaining olive oil as needed to form into desirable consistency. Sauce can be kept refrigerated for a few days if stored in a jar with a tight fitting lid. If doing this add a small amount of olive oil to pesto in jar to top off sauce with a thin layer of film while storing. Pesto however is best if used immediately.

Approx. 350 calories per serving
7g protein, 36g fat, 2g carbohydrates,
10mg cholesterol, 233mg sodium, 0 fiber

SPICY GARLICKY PESTO SAUCE (Use as a pasta sauce or a pizza sauce)

Ingredients: Makes 4 servings

1/4 cup extra- virgin olive oil
4 cloves garlic, chopped
1/4 teaspoon red hot pepper flakes
Salt and pepper to taste

In a medium sized skillet over medium heat, warm olive oil. Add garlic and sauté until translucent. Add hot pepper flakes and simmer on very low heat for 3-5 minutes. Serve with your favorite pasta. Garnish with grated cheese if desired.

> **Approx. 134 calories per serving**
> **0 protein, 14g fat, 1 g carbohydrates,**
> **0 cholesterol, 0 sodium, 0 fiber**

ANCHOVY AND GARLIC SAUCE (use for pasta or pizza)

Ingredients: Makes 4 servings

6 tablespoons extra-virgin olive oil + oil from anchovies
6 cloves fresh garlic, pressed
2 oz. tin of anchovy fillets packed in oil, drained and chopped
Red hot pepper flakes to taste
2 tablespoons cilantro, finely chopped
6 tablespoons freshly grated Romano cheese
Salt and freshly ground pepper to taste

Combine oil and garlic in a skillet over medium heat and cook about 1-2 minutes. Add anchovies, cook about 30 seconds and remove from heat. Add hot pepper flakes and cilantro. Serve with choice of Pasta or use as pizza sauce. Add salt and pepper as desired.

> *Approx. 253 calories per serving*
> *6g protein, 25g fat, 1g carbohydrates,*
> *18mg cholesterol, 517mg sodium, 0 fiber*

SUNDRIED TOMATO PESTO
(Use as a pasta sauce or as a pizza sauce)

Ingredients: Makes 2 cups

1 cup sundried tomatoes
2 cups boiling water
1/4 cup plus 1/2 tablespoon extra-virgin olive oil
5 cloves garlic
1/4 cup pine nuts
1/2 cup fresh basil
1/2 cup Italian parsley

Combine boiling water and sundried tomatoes, let stand till tomatoes soften, about 10-15 minutes. Drain and reserve 1 cup of liquid. In a medium skillet heat 1/2 tablespoon oil over medium-high heat. Add garlic and sauté, stirring often for about 1 minute. Remove from heat. Process tomatoes, reserved liquid, pine nuts, basil, parsley and remaining 1/4 cup olive oil and garlic.

> *Approx. 70 calories per 2 tablespoons*
> *2g protein, 6g fat, 3g carbohydrates,*
> *0 cholesterol, 72mg sodium, 1g fiber*

RED CLAM SAUCE (Use as a pasta sauce)

Ingredients: Makes 4 servings

1/2 cup white wine
3 cloves garlic, crushed
48 small hard shell clams
1 onion, chopped
2 tablespoons extra-virgin olive oil
2 cups diced plum tomatoes
Salt and pepper to taste
1 teaspoon chopped parsley

In a large pot, cook wine, garlic and clams in small amount of water until shells open. Remove clams from shells. In a skillet add onion to heated olive oil and sauté. Add diced tomatoes, season and cook for 8 minutes. Add clams in their juices and cook for another 2-3 minutes. Serve over pasta and garnish with parsley.

> *Approx. (sauce only) 139 calories per serving*
> *14g protein, 1g fat, 8g carbohydrates,*
> *37mg cholesterol, 298mg sodium, 2g fiber*

SARDINE PASTA SAUCE

Ingredients: Makes 4 servings

1/3 cup black olives, pitted and chopped (like Kalamata or Nicoise)
1 tin of sardines packed in olive oil
2 cloves fresh garlic, pressed
Red hot pepper flakes to taste
1/4 cup extra-virgin olive oil
1/4 cup finely chopped cilantro
Salt and pepper to taste

Combine all the ingredients and mix until sardines are broken into small pieces. Toss with cooked pasta of choice with, add salt and pepper to taste and serve.

> *Approx. 227 calories per serving*
> *5g protein, 22g fat, 1g carbohydrate,*
> *0 cholesterol, 315mg sodium, 0 fiber*

SPICY PISTACHIO PESTO *(great fish topper)*

Ingredients: Makes 4 servings

1/2 small hot cherry pepper, seeded
3 cloves garlic, peeled
2 roasted red peppers
1/4 cup shelled pistachios, roasted
1/3 cup extra-virgin olive oil
1/4 cup fresh grated Parmesan cheese
Salt and pepper to taste

In a food processor combine hot peppers, garlic, red peppers and pistachios. Season with salt and pepper; pulse while adding olive oil a little at a time, until it forms a smooth consistency. Transfer to a bowl and blend in cheese.

> *Approx. 255 calories per serving*
> *4g protein, 24g fat, 5g carbohydrates,*
> *6mg cholesterol, 101mg sodium, 1g fiber*

LEMON DRESSING

Ingredients: Makes about 1/2 cup of dressing (1 tablespoon per serving)

1/4 cup extra-virgin olive oil
1/4 cup fresh squeezed lemon juice
1 medium garlic clove, crushed to a paste
1 pinch salt
Fresh ground black pepper to taste

Combine all ingredients in a bowl and mix well.

> *Approx. 71 calories per tablespoon*
> *0 protein, 7g fat, 1g carbohydrate,*
> *0 cholesterol, 0 sodium, 0 fiber*

SKORDALIA

Greek garlic topping, great for fish or chicken, broccoli and cauliflower

Ingredients: Makes 2 1/2 cups

3 slices bread, crust removed
1 cup blanched almonds, finely chopped
6 cloves garlic, chopped fine
Salt to taste
3 tablespoons fresh lemon juice
3/4 cup extra-virgin olive oil

In a food processor, using a metal blade chop bread into pieces. Add ground almonds, garlic and salt and continue processing to form a paste. Add lemon juice and mix well. Add olive oil a few drops at a time, as you are processing until mixture becomes thick and creamy. Continue adding oil until mixture is light and fluffy. Transfer to serving bowl and serve.

PISTACHIO PESTO SALAD DRESSING

Ingredients: Makes 4 servings

3 cloves garlic, peeled
2 roasted red peppers
1/4 cup shelled pistachios, roasted
1/3 cup extra-virgin olive oil
1/4 cup fresh grated parmesan cheese
Salt and pepper to taste

In a food processor combine garlic, roasted peppers and pistachios. Season with salt and pepper; and process adding olive oil a little at a time, until it forms a smooth consistency. Transfer to a bowl and blend in cheese.

> *Approx. 255 calories per serving*
> *4g protein, 24g fat, 5g carbohydrates,*
> *6mg cholesterol, 101mg sodium, 1g fiber*

SICILIAN DRESSING

Great topping for fish or as a salad dressing

Ingredients: Makes about 1 cup dressing sauce

1/4 cup water
2/3 cup extra-virgin olive oil
Juice from 1 lemon
2 cloves garlic, sliced
1/2 cup fresh parsley, chopped
1 teaspoon oregano

Scald water. Add olive oil to a bowl, pour in scalded water and beat. Add lemon juice, garlic, parsley and oregano and beat again until well mixed. Place mixture in a double boiler and cook for additional 5 minutes, stirring constantly. Use as fish topper or let cool and serve over salad.

Approx. 130 calories per tablespoon
0 protein, 14g fat, 0 carbohydrates,
0 cholesterol, 0 sodium, 0 fiber

Appendix

OLIVE OIL

T he history of the olive has been passed down through generations in myths and legends and in books about love and war and other great events in history. Buying olive oil can be both exciting and confusing because of the vast variety of oils available in supermarkets, and specialty food markets. There are virgin-oils and pure-oils throughout the Mediterranean basin. There are emerald green colored oils and golden oils. Oils come bottled in different sizes and shapes, from exquisite glass bottles to metal tins and even plastic containers. So how does one start to make a selection?

Olive oils range from a pale yellow color to a deep cloudy green. One can easily assume that the latter is from green barely ripe olives. If an olive oil appears green in color it is often an indication that the oil has a wonderful intensely fresh fruity taste. Yellow oil, however usually means that the olives were picked late in the season, when black and ripe. The later picked olives usually produce sweeter, rounder flavored oil. However, if an oil smells or tastes rancid it usually indicates that it has been exposed to sunlight or another source of light, reducing the delicate aromatic qualities and vitamin E content of the oil. When selecting an oil look for the harvest date on the bottle. No olive oil improves with age, so it should not be more than eighteen months old. Olive oil far exceeds the health benefits of other oils, butters, margarines or lard; it should be used to replace these items not in conjunction with them.

There are various grades of olive oil:
- Extra-virgin: obtained from the first pressing of the olives
- Fine virgin: the oil comes from the second pressing of the olives
- Refined oil: the oil is created by using chemicals to extract the oil from the olives
- Pure oil: a blend of refined and virgin olive oils

Scientific studies have demonstrated the advantage of using virgin rather than refined olive oil since virgin olive oil has more anti-oxidant properties and tends to raise the good HDL cholesterol better than refined olive oil. People with high cholesterol who replace saturated fat in their diet with olive oil decrease their total cholesterol and bad LDL cholesterol.

Mediterraneans grow up with the taste of their local oil ingrained in their senses. When you consume a local olive oil, the very essence of its origin bathes your taste buds and from this, one can almost envision the soil and the tree that produced its fruit. An excellent olive oil can range from thirty to forty dollars or as high as eighty dollars a bottle, much like an expensive bottle of wine of corresponding quality

When you buy olive oil consider how you will use it. If you want to make a pasta sizzle, a young, peppery Tuscan oil might be the best. Whereas a good cured full-bodied oil would be appropriate for a traditional Greek salad made of the best quality tomatoes and finest feta available. However if you want a hint of olive oil with a background flavor then, a light fruity olive oil, perhaps one from Liguria or Provence that adds a layer of flavor but does not stand out would be best.

Artisanal oils are ones that are not really pressed but rather are made by big industrial state-of-the-art machinery, where the water of the olive, called vegetable water, is spun off from the oil, much like cream is spun off of milk. Artisanal oils are found in most supermarkets. These bulk oils are a mixture of oils from Italy, Spain, Tunisia, Greece, and even Turkey. They are your everyday olive oils that most Americans are familiar with. They are not the olive oils of grand distinction and may not be the oils one would like to use in a special meal.

A few favorite quality extra-virgin olive oils that are available in most specialty markets in the United States:

Italy:

Castello di Ama (Tuscany)
Gemini (Tuscan and Sicilian blend)
Ardoino (Liguria)
Grandverde Colanna (Central Italy)
Capezzana (Tuscany)
Badia a Coltibuono (Tuscany)
Trevi Umbro (Umbria)
Raineri (Liguria)
La Giara (Calabria- Southern Italy)

Greece:

Greek Gold Organic (Mani peninsula)
Kolymvari (Crete)
Kydonia (Crete)

Spanish:

Lerda (Catalonia)
Almazara (Murcia)
Nunez de Prado (Andalusia)

French:

M.Bellon's Moulin de Bedarrides (Provence)

California:

B.R. Cohen Sonoma Estate
Davero
Frantoio Proprietor's Select
Harrison Olio d'Oro
"O" Olive Oil
Sciabica & Sons Ascalano Oil

Bulk Oils- available in most supermarkets in the United States

Colavita
Sasso
Bertolli
Lucini
Bellino

BEANS

Beans (legumes) are high in complex carbohydrates, amino acids, fiber, iron, and folic acid. They contain little to no fat and no cholesterol however they do contain an abundance of soluble fiber, which benefits our hearts by lowering cholesterol levels. They are also an excellent low-fat source of protein as well as a source of complex carbohydrates. In the Mediterranean, legumes are eaten almost every day as part of a main meal. They could be served cold or be served as a main dish or as part of a stew or perhaps a dip, to be scooped up with bread or vegetables. There are so many delicious ways in which they can be served. There are a few general rules about buying beans. Buy only beans that are smooth and bright in color. Beans are old if they appear cracked, dull and or wrinkled. The older the bean, the longer the cooking time needed. One (1) cup of dry beans equals 2-2 1/2 cups of cooked beans. Most dried beans must be soaked before they are cooked. The only exception is lentils. There are two methods used for soaking beans, the power soak method or the long soak method.

- Power soaking is a method whereby the dried beans are boiled in water for about 3 minutes then covered and set aside for 2 to 4 hours. After 4 hours the water is drained off and discarded and the beans are rinsed under fresh running water. The beans are then returned to a heavy bottomed pot, covered with fresh water and cooked as per package directions.
- Long soak method requires the beans to be soaked for 8 hours or more. After the required soaking time the water covering the beans is also discarded. As with the power method, the beans are rinsed under fresh water then returned to a heavy bottomed pot with fresh water and cooked as per package directions.

For either method of soaking, you can test a bean for adequate soaking simply by cutting the bean in half to check its color. If the center is opaque in color, then soak them longer.

Here are a few hints for basic bean seasoning. Cook beans from the start with the following basic seasonings: chopped onions, garlic cloves, bay leaves, and cumin. You can add other spices to your liking but wait until the beans are almost done before adding major seasonings. Adding spices too soon can cause them to break down and disappear. A bean is fully cooked when it can be mashed with a fork.

Humble bean dishes are served everywhere in the Mediterranean as a first course or even as the main dish. Hearty bean soups are a staple all around the Mediterranean, made with grains and an abundance of vegetables. On wintry days, throughout the countryside, the delicious aroma of hearty bean soups that have been simmering for days can be smelled everywhere.

Some of the more popular beans used in the Mediterranean include:

Cannellini Beans: Probably one of the most popular beans used in cuisines of central Italy. A little white kidney-shaped bean high in protein. They are great in soups and salads as well as by themselves with just a little olive oil drizzled over them. Soaking time is about 11/2 hours (ratio of 1 cup of beans to 3 cups of water). One half cup of cooked cannellini beans is roughly 100 calories.

Fava Beans (white or brown): Also called broad beans, go back almost to the beginning of Mediterranean agriculture. They have tough outer skins (which is usually discarded after soaking) and a sweet nutty flavored inner texture and taste. They are great in soups and salads and are often used for dips and paté. Soaking time is about 3 hours (ratio of 1 cup of beans to 4 cups of water). One half cup of fava beans is roughly 93 calories.

Chickpeas or Garbanzos: These too are Old World beans with a long history in Mediterranean agriculture. In North African regions they are used to make hummus. They are an excellent source of protein and iron. Soaking time is about 3 hours (ratio of 1 cup of beans to 4 cups of water). One half cup of cooked chickpeas is roughly 130 calories.

Great Northern Beans: Are classified in the family of white beans and similar in flavor to the navy bean, which is smaller in size. They do well in many dishes also in an oil and vinegar marinade. Soaking time is about 2 hours (ratio of 1 cup of beans to 3 cups of water). One half cup of cooked great northern is roughly 100 calories.

Navy Beans: Also of the white bean family. They are great in soups and salads and stand alone well just in a vinegar and oil marinade. Soaking time is about 2 1/2 hours (ratio of 1 cup of beans to 4 cups of water). On half cup of cooked navy beans is roughly 130 calories.

Lentils: brown, red or green lentils are a stable in many Mediterranean cuisines. Never substitute Indian lentils in a Mediterranean dish, they are meant to disintegrate into a thick sauce upon cooking. In Mediterranean cuisine, the opposite effect is desired. In these dishes they are meant to remain intact. Brown and green lentils do well in salads where as red ones are better suited for pate and soups. No soaking is required.

Favorite spices used in France and Italy include rosemary, fennel, sage, caraway, tarragon and marjoram. Lighter spices often include combinations of bay leaves, garlic, oregano, parsley, thyme and dill. Often a dash of balsamic vinegar or a drizzle of a fruity olive oil is added. Lemon juice or even tomatoes and cheese are sometimes included. In the Middle Eastern countries stronger spices such as cumin, cinnamon, mint and coriander prevail and lighter combinations of garlic, ginger, nutmeg, fresh pepper, marjoram, parsley, cilantro, saffron, paprika or turmeric are mixed together.

Flatulence can be a major problem for some people when consuming beans. Never use the same water that the beans have been soaking in to also cook the beans. Always discard the soaking water, rinse beans and cook them in fresh water. This will help prevent the problem of flatulence and even help to avoid it completely.

GRAINS

Grains, which make up the foundation of the Mediterranean diet, appear at almost every meal, in one form or the other. Grains can take the form of rice, wheat (to make bread, pasta, couscous or bulgur) or polenta. Grains, also provide the bulk of protein and many of the calories in the Mediterranean diet and are a perfect energy source in the form of complex carbohydrates.

RICE

In the Mediterranean diet, rice is as popular as fine wheat flour, and in some regions it's a first choice. World-wide it is the most consumed food, eaten by millions every day. In the regions of the western Mediterranean, dishes like risotto and paella have evolved. In Greece, Turkey, and the Levant, long-grain rice, originally from India and Persia, is preferred since they make a better pilaf. Long-grain rice cooks up dry and fluffy whereas short-grains are more tender and sticky. Brown rice, unquestionably a healthier product, is not often used in the Mediterranean except by macrobiotics.

Secrets for cooking rice successfully vary. The general ratio for most rice is 1 cup of rice to 1-1/2 or 2 cups of water. Put your rice in a heavy pot with water and salt and cover with a tight fitting lid, bring to a boil, then reduce heat to medium-low and let simmer for 1 hour, or until water is completely absorbed. Finally, when the time is up, keep the pot covered tightly for another 10 minutes before serving.

WHEAT

Wheat is one of the cornerstones of the Mediterranean diet. It is seen in the form of bread, pasta, couscous or bulgur. There are many types of wheat ranging from very soft wheat (Triticum aestivum) to very hard wheat (Triticum durum). The terms soft and hard do not refer to the texture of the wheat but the protein content of the wheat. Hard wheat is generally both higher in protein and gluten which is needed for bread making. Durum hard grain, is the hardest wheat grown, and is usually milled into semolina. It is the hardest of all wheat and although it is a soft creamy yellow, its texture is coarser than regular wheat flour.

Semolina flour therefore comes from the heart of durum wheat. Semolina is a golden grain that has a higher protein and gluten content and is used almost exclusively for pasta production; it is also used to make couscous and home-made breads in Morocco. Couscous is made from pre-cooked semolina flour that is actually granules of cracked durum wheat with a tawny yellow color and a silken light texture. The creamy, silky golden flour also makes wonderful bread, but it does need to be kneaded for a long time. It can be used alone but is often combined with unbleached or all-purpose flour for bread making. Soft wheat (Triticum aestivum) is most often used for commercial pizza dough and pastries.

The best all-purpose flour is a blend of hard and soft wheat that are unbleached and unbromated. Unbleached means that the flour has not been treated with chemicals such as chlorine or peroxide to make it whiter. Most health food stores carry at least one unbleached and unbromated type of all-purpose flour. A flours performance, flavor and nutrition are greatly affected by the type of mill that grinds the grain.

Whole wheat flour contains the whole wheat berry. The amount of husk and wheat germ retained varies depending upon how it is milled. Stone-ground mills produce the best flour. This is because this milling process does not overheat the flour, it flakes layers off the grain, resulting in more of the nutrients being retained in the flour. Whole wheat flour is stone-ground.

All wheat flour contains varying levels of gluten. Gluten is the natural protein derived from wheat. Gluten is the substance in wheat that is responsible for the stretchiness of dough.

PASTA

Pasta comes in many shapes, flavors and textures, however they all share the same basic ingredients, flour and water. The best industrial pasta is made from semolina flour, because it absorbs much less water than other flours. Semolina is the flour ground from the heart (or endosperm) of durum wheat, the hardest of all wheats. The best pastas list durum wheat flour or semolina in their ingredients. Those imported from Italy are usually the best because of their fine quality semolina. One pound of pasta generally feeds 6 people as an appetizer and 4 people as a main course. Two ounces of uncooked pasta generally equals 1 cup of cooked pasta. Generally pureed, creamy or clinging sauces are best served with thin strands of pasta like spaghetti, fettuccine, cappellini or linguine pastas that will allow the sauce to flow evenly over the noodle. Thinner, runnier sauces are better held by pastas that have twisted or curled shapes that trap the liquid so that the sauce coats the pasta rather than the plate. Whereas chunky sauces go best with chunky pastas, pastas that contain an opening, like elbow macaroni or shell pastas. Tiny pastas like Orzo are great with a little olive oil and herbs whereas rich sauces tend to overwhelm them.

Tips for cooking pasta:

Use 3 quarts of rapidly boiling water for 1/2 pound of pasta and (4) quarts for (1) pound of pasta. Make sure your pot is large and roomy. You should salt the water before adding pasta. Generally use 1 teaspoon of salt per 1/2 pound of pasta. Add pasta to boiling water, do not stir noodles that stick to the bottom of the pot but gently lift them with a fork. Check pasta at 2-4 minutes for thin pasta and 8-10 minutes for denser pasta. When cooked, drain pasta but do not rinse. This keeps the pasta moist and helps the sauces to stick. Add sauce immediately and serve. If not ready to serve, toss pasta with 1-2 tablespoons of olive oil to prevent pasta from sticking. If serving as a pasta salad, put dressing on hot noodles immediately to let it sink in. If pasta is going to be cooked further, such as in a baked dish, undercook it slightly when boiling the pasta. This is called al dente. Because pastas come in many shapes and flavors, their caloric value per cup varies greatly.

Pasta comes in a variety of shapes. Listed below are just a few examples:

Spaghetti in Italian means "a length of cord". All of the spaghetti family consists of long, thin round noodles. They therefore lend themselves to lightly sauced dishes. Some of the different types of spaghetti are:
- Capellini - also known as angel hair
- Spaghettini - little lengths of cord
- Vermicelli - a very thin, short round noodle
- Fusilli Bucati - a twisted or spiral shaped spaghetti.

Fettuccine in Italian means "small ribbon". This family of pasta is long and flat and ranges from 1/16 of an inch to 3 inches. The thinner of these pastas, linguine and tagliatelle, work well with lighter sauces. Some other different types of black ribbon pastas are:
- Linguini - a long flat pasta thinner in width than fettuccine
- Tagliatelle - a flat pasta wider than linguini but smaller than fettuccine
- Lasagna - a curly or plain edged flat pasta 2-3 inches wide

Macaroni are tubular pastas. They can be long or short ribbed or grooved. These pastas lend themselves to thick chunky meat or vegetable sauces. Examples of these pastas are:
- Penne - a 2 inch long and smooth tubular pasta
- Rigatoni - a larger tubular pasta with groves on the outside
- Ziti - a tubular pasta either straight or slightly curved and can be either smoothed or grooved on the outside

Small pastas are great for soups. The smaller ones such as alphabet noodles and pastina are best in light brothy soups. Thicker soups do well with Ditalini and Tubetti noodles. Other types of small pastas include Orzo which are rice shaped, Anellini that look like tiny rings and Tubettini which are slightly larger than Tubetti.

Miscellaneous noodles like elbow, ties, shells and other various decorative shapes. These pastas are great with heavy cheese sauces or in casseroles. The large shells or tubular sauces are great stuffed. Examples of these pastas are:
- Cannelloni - which are very large tubular shaped noodles
- Cavatelli shells - which are small and narrow
- Conchiglie - a medium sized shell
- Sarsalla - also called the bow tie
- Gnocchi shells - are shaped much like the Cavatelli shell but are thicker and made from a potato dough
- Manicotti - large tubular noodles like Cannelloni
- Ravioli - hollow square pasta often stuffed with cheeses, ground

meat, vegetables or seafood.

There are many high quality brand pastas available in this country. The key to keeping pasta a healthy low fat food is to use whole wheat pasta and not to top any pasta dish with rich fatty sauces.

COUSCOUS

What pasta is to the Italians and rice is to the Chinese, couscous is to the countries of Morocco, Algeria and Tunisia. Couscous is a mainstay in these countries. When entering a kitchen during meal time it would be quite common to see a steaming platter of couscous, topped with vegetables, meat or fish, and broth. Couscous is often used with only vegetables and perhaps a cheese (goat cheese) and or nuts. Meat is usually served only once a week and is usually lamb, chicken, or pork. Couscous is used to make appetizers, soups, salads, main course dishes and even desserts.

Couscous is made from wheat, which has been an essential part of the Mediterranean diet since time immemorial. Durum wheat, the hardest form of wheat is best suited for the production of couscous. It is low in starch and high in protein content. The wheat is milled in its coarsest form called "semolina". It is then rolled into thin strands, crumbled into tiny pieces, steamed and dried. It is unlike pasta since it is not kneaded during the semolina-water mixture stage. The word "couscous" refers both to the dry durum wheat semolina product as well as to the popular prepared dish in which it is the principal ingredient.

The coarsest and largest size couscous is used primarily for soups. The medium-sized, that which is mostly seen here in the United States, have and all- purpose application, whereas the tiny or ant sized ones are reserved for special dishes and desserts.

For the sake of convenience only pre-steamed couscous, that is available in the United States, is used. Pre-steamed couscous greatly reduces the final cooking time for a dish, since it takes only fifteen minutes in boiling liquid until it is ready to serve.

BULGUR

Bulgur is made by cracking parboiled whole wheat kernels and drying them. Parboiling is simply boiling the kernel until it is partially cooked. Bulgur wheat does not need to be cooked further, but should be soaked in warm water for 20-30 minutes to soften before using. It is commonly used in salad preparations but most often used to make Tabbouleh. Bulgur can also be used to make pilaf, however you should not soak it before using it in a pilaf recipe.

POLENTA

Polenta is a gluten-free coarsely-ground cornmeal, either white or yellow in color, rather like semolina in appearance, and is made from maize. The best polenta is stone-ground cornmeal where the whole grain is used, including the germ. It is a favorite dish in northern Italy where it is cooked in water and then eaten with a drizzle of olive oil and a sprinkle of Parmesan cheese or with tomato sauce. It is a traditional dish and often replaces rice, pasta or potatoes.

GLOSSARY

Al dente: Italian for pasta cooked slightly resistant to the bite.

All-purpose flour: is a blend of soft and hard wheat. The best type is unbleached.

Antioxidants: compounds that may have the potential to prevent numerous diseases because they interfere with the cellular destruction caused by free-radicals. Antioxidants wander through the body searching out and destroying free-radicals.

Basil: a very aromatic herb with a sweet, mildly pungent flavor. A favorite and widely used spice in Italy.

Bay leaf: The greener the leaf the more flavor it has. Great in soups, meat dishes and sauces.

Bruschetta: Crusty slices of bread drenched with extra-virgin olive oil and rubbed with generous amounts of garlic and grilled or toasted on both sides.

Bulgur: whole-wheat kernels that are steamed, dried and crushed. Bulgur comes in three grades, coarse, medium and fine. They have a tender chewy consistency. The coarser size is best for pilaf while the medium size is good for Tabbouleh.

Calorie: a unit of heat energy that expresses the energy exchanges of the body and the potential energy values of food.

Carbohydrates: sources of food energy either in the form of complex carbohydrates or simple carbohydrates.

Cayenne: The dried and powdered fruit of the red hot pepper. It is much like paprika in appearance and is used in small amounts to give a fiery kick to many dishes.

Cholesterol: type of fat derived from animal sources. Cholesterol is transported through the body by carriers called lipoproteins. Excessive amounts of cholesterol circulating in the blood can build up on artery walls and eventually lead to heart attack and stroke

Cilantro: also known as coriander or Chinese parsley.

Complex carbohydrates: energy-yielding nutrients which provide the most efficient fuel source for the body. Complex carbohydrates metabolize more slowly than simple carbohydrates providing the body with energy over a longer period of time. Examples of complex carbohydrates are legumes, vegetables and whole grains.

Cornmeal: is either white or yellow however yellow is more typical. It has a grainy texture and sweet taste. In Italy cornmeal is called polenta.

Couscous: is not a distinct grain but rather a type of pasta made from hard semolina wheat and water. What rice is to the Chinese, couscous is to the lands of Morocco, Algeria and Tunisia. Couscous is now available in an instant form which just needs to be covered with boiling water.

Crostini: thinner slices of crusty bread, baked in an oven at 350 degrees F., until golden in color, and rubbed with garlic and drenched in extra-virgin olive oil.

Cumin: a dried, slightly bitter fruit that is part of the parsley family. It has a strong scent and flavor.

Dietary Fiber: comes from the walls of plants. They are the parts of fruits and vegetables and whole grains that are not digested or absorbed by the body. There are two types of dietary fiber, soluble and insoluble.

Insoluble fibers add bulk to stools and help you fell satiated. Soluble fiber forms a jell-like mass around food parts and helps to prevent the absorption of cholesterol by promoting its excretion.

Durum Flour: comes from the hardest kind of wheat; it is ground from durum wheat. Durum flour is very fine flour and is very high in gluten content.

Farro: is an ancient strain of soft wheat. In Tuscany it is often served as a whole-grain in soups and stews.

Fat: one of three main classes of nutrients that provide energy to the body. Fats are either saturated or unsaturated (monounsaturated and polyunsaturated).

Feta cheese: is made from pasteurized sheep's or goat's milk.

Focaccia: an Italian oven baked round or rectangular bread filled with herbs, onions, spices and often an array of vegetables.

Free radicals: unstable products of metabolism. They react with oxygen creating oxidation which has a destructive effect on the cells DNA. The damaged DNA causes a cascading effect of not only suppressing our immune system but has also been implicated in the development of many diseases such as heart disease, cancer and other chronic illnesses.

Garlic: has beneficial effects on blood pressure, cholesterol and other risk factors. The flavor can be mild or strong depending on how it is sliced or chopped. The longer it is cooked the milder the flavor becomes.

Gluten: a protein substance (esp. of wheat flour) that gives cohesiveness to dough.

Harissa, hareesa or hreesa: fiery hot paste made by pounding together red chili peppers, spices, and olive oil. It is used to season couscous and many North African dishes.

Italian frittatas: are savory omelets, cooked into a thick cake brimming with potatoes and onions or other vegetables. It is most delicious when served warm from the oven.

Kesera Sesame Bread: A Moroccan type of round flat bread that is slightly crunchy on the outside and chewy on the inside. Great for dipping in soups or with stews.

Kesra: Is a dense round loaf of bread predominately seen in the Northwestern African regions of Morocco, Algeria and Tunisia. Kesra is flavored with whole aniseeds or sesame seeds.

Khubz: pita bread. The Arabs eat bread with every meal. They use it to scoop up sauces, dips, yogurts and liquids or pita cut in half can be filled with Shish Kabobs, falafel or salads. They consider bread to be a divine gift from God.

Lavosh: A very crispy flat Egyptian bread.

Mazza: An array of appetizers and small dishes.

Mediterranean Crusty-Country bread: a favorite hearty slightly sour crusty bread consumed throughout France, Italy, Spain and Portugal.

Mint: has a strong sweet aroma and is available fresh or dried. Also great as a garnish.

Monounsaturated fat: is a naturally occurring heart-healthy fat found in plant foods. Research has found that monounsaturated fats actually play an important role in helping to prevent the risk of heart disease and cancers. It is felt that it generally helps to maintain or raise the good cholesterol (HDL) while decreasing bad (LDL) cholesterol. A few examples of foods high in monounsaturated fats are nuts, olives, olive oil and avocados.

Mozzarella: is a soft spongy white cheese with a slightly sour flavor.

Obesity: A condition whereby a person exceeds the healthy weight for his or her height and body composition by 20% or more. The BMI or body mass index is used to define obesity. The BMI categories:
< 18.5 underweight
18.5 – 24.9 normal weight
25 – 29.9 overweight
> 30 obesity

Oregano: a very popular Italian herb, closely related to marjoram.

Paella: a variable Spanish rice dish often containing chicken, mussels, whitefish, peas, and rice and flavored with saffron, salt, pepper, and pimiento.

Parmesan cheese: is a hard cheese made from semi-skimmed unpasteurized cow's milk.

Parsley: One of the most commonly used herbs. It adds both flavor and color to many dishes.

Pecorino: is a sheep's milk cheese. It is recently becoming more available in finer cheese shops here in the United States.

Pesto: The word comes from the Italian verb pestare, which means to pound. It was often handmade using a mortal and pestle to grind the herbs leaving a wonderful coarseness lending itself to a great taste and texture. It was said that this assertive green sauce was a traditional basil sauce favorite of Genoese sailors. In Italy, Italians are discreet with pesto, a little of this rich and highly flavored sauce goes a long way. Today, pre-made pesto sauces are available in most markets. The fresh pesto in tubs usually has more flavor then the jar varieties, however nothing is as good as home-made.

Pistou: is a pounded pesto like sauce made of nuts, olive oil, garlic and basil. It is unique to the Mediterranean region in France. It adds both body and herbaceous flavor to soups and stews.

Pita bread: a flat, round, hollow bread common to the cuisines of Africa and the Middle East.

Polenta: is just cornmeal in a coarser texture. Pre-cooked instant polenta is now available in most markets, but does not taste as good as home-made polenta.

Polyunsaturated fat: is an unsaturated fat found in foods like corn, sunflower and safflower oils.

Ratatouille: a vegetable casserole of tomatoes, eggplant, green peppers, zucchini, onions, and seasonings.

Risotto: an Italian rice dish made with butter, chopped onion, stock or wine, and parmesan cheese. Meats or seafood and vegetables may also be added.

Saffron: Dried yellow crocus native to the Mediterranean with a strong yellow color and a delicate flavor used in many dishes. A rather expensive spice.

Saturated fat: type of fat found in animal foods such as red meat, poultry and dairy products, such as butter and whole milk. Other foods high in saturated fats include tropical cooking oils such as palm and coconut oils. High intakes of saturated fats have been linked to cardiovascular disease and cancer.

Semolina: roughly ground durum wheat used to make pasta and bread. It is technically not a grain but a nutritive tissue of durum wheat, the hardest of all wheat. It is traditionally used to make pasta.

Simple carbohydrates: sugars which are quickly absorbed into the blood stream providing an immediate source of energy. Food sources like candy and soda are good examples of simple carbohydrates.

Soft and hard (wheat): refers not just to the texture of the wheat but also to the protein content. Most hard wheat is higher in protein and higher in the gluten, which is necessary for bread making.

Tahini: a paste made from crushed sesame seeds.

Tapas: Spanish appetizers, often called the "Little Dishes of Spain."

Trans-fats: type of fat found in stick margarine and vegetable shortening and any food product that lists hydrogenated oils as part of its ingredients. The consumption of food products containing trans-fats has been linked with the development of heart disease, diabetes, obesity and cancer.

Turmeric: is a member of the ginger family. It is a rich yellow spice with flavoring similar to saffron and less expensive than saffron. Often used instead of saffron in many dishes.

Whole-wheat flour: is dark whole-grain flour that has not had the bran and germ milled out of it. Some whole-wheat are coarser than others. The best stone-ground has a nutty wholesome flavor.

Whole-wheat pastry flour: is made from softer wheat and is more finely milled than whole-wheat flour. In Italy it is used to make pizza and other pastries.

INDEX

MAIN DISHES 132

SIDE DISHES 180

OMELETS or FRITTATAS 123

PIZZA 107

PIZZA SAUCES 116

PIZZA CRUST 120

WRAPS and SANDWICHES 211

Smoked fish and roasted pepper sandwich, 221

BREADS 222

Mediterranean crusty country bread, 223
Focaccia, 224
Egyptian Khutz (pita bread), 225
Lavosh, 226
Sesame bread (Kersa), 227

APPETIZERS, DIPS and SNACKS 248

Stuffed grape leaves (Dolmas), 248
Marinated olives, 250
Tomato and garlic topping for bruschette, 251
Tomato and fresh cheese bruschette topping, 252
Roasted garlic, 253
Quick garlic bruschette, 253
Italian crostini, 254
Chilled avocado dip, 255
Hummus dip (chickpeas), 256
Greek bean dip, 257
Greek feta and walnut dip, 258
Skordalia, 259
Herb cucumber yogurt dip, 260
Roasted pepper dip, 261
Toasted Tahini dip, 262
Hummus with Tahini dip, 263

SPICES, SAUCES and DRESSINGS 264

SPICES

SAUCES

DRESSINGS

DESSERTS 228

THE 10 COMMANDMENTS FOR A HEART- HEALTHY MEDITERRANEAN DIET & LIFESTYLE

1 – Heart – healthy diet:

- Fresh fruits and vegetables
- Whole grains
- Nuts
- Beans
- Soy protein
- Fish
- Low fat yogurt and cheese
- Plant sterol vegetable spreads

2 – Consume extra-virgin olive oil

3 – Drink 6 to 8 glasses of water per day

4 – Wine with meals. Avoid excessive alcohol consumption.

5 – Relaxation (esp. after meals)

6 – Exercise – minimum 30 minutes per day

7 – Limit portion size

8 – Avoid processed or refined foods

9 – Read food labels – avoid saturated fats and trans-fats

10 – Laugh, smile and enjoy life!